CHAPTEl
About Adrenal Glands & Hc. ιιone Production

Before we get to the good things to help you heal Adrenal Fatigue naturally, it's vital to first apprehend what the adrenal glands are, how they paintings, and what function they play in a healthy-functioning frame. It's a touch intensive, however endure with me. This will assist you higher apprehend why and the way a number of the remedies I propose paintings.

Adrenal glands are a key element of what's known as the HPA Axis: the hypothalamus, pituitary, and the adrenal glands. These 3 glands paintings collectively in a remarks loop to manipulate and alter metabolism and strength ranges, libido, immune system, temper and pressure reaction.

Hypothalamus
The hypothalamus, positioned deep withinside the forebrain, produces and secretes the hormone "corticotrophin-freeing factor", or CRF, in reaction to pressure. The greater pressure, the greater CRF is generated through the hypothalamus.

Pituitary
The pituitary sits beneath the hypothalamus. As the hypothalamus secretes CRF, it stimulates the pituitary to launch adrenocorticotropic hormone (ACTH), which travels to the adrenals and kidneys.

Adrenals
The adrenals are walnut-sized glands positioned simply above every of the kidneys and that they play a massive function on your normal wellbeing. *(The root of the word "adrenal" comes from the Latin "ad", or near, and "renes", that's kidney.) They reply to the messages from the pituitary through generating hormones or chemical compounds that alter the metabolism*, infection and immune reaction.

Each adrenal gland is produced from awesome parts, with awesome features.

Adrenal Cortex
This is the outer layer, or shell, of the gland. Its task is to provide hormones that have an effect on metabolism and different chemical compounds

withinside the blood.

Cortisol
Cortisol is one of the stars of the glucocorticoid family. Cortisol is well-known for triggering our bodily pressure reaction to depression, anxiety, and extra exercise, loss of sleep or trauma. Cortisol stimulates norepinephrine, every now and then known as noradrenaline, to position the frame into "combat or flight" mode. I will cope with greater approximately cortisol in a moment.

Aldosterone
Aldosterone regulates potassium and sodium ranges, and allows to hold blood stress and blood volume.

Androgenic Steroids (Androgen Hormones)
The androgenic hormones, along with DHEA (dehydroepiandrosterone), produced withinside the adrenal cortex are transformed into woman hormones (estrogen) or male hormones (androgens and testosterone), and they may be additionally produced some place else withinside the frame in large quantities.

Adrenal Medulla
This internal center of the adrenal gland is chargeable for generating the hormones that assist us address emotional and bodily pressure.

Epinephrine (Adrenaline)
Epinephrine enables blood glide to the muscle groups and the mind, allows convert glycogen to glucose withinside the liver, and will increase each the coronary heart price and the pressure of coronary heart contractions.

Norepinephrine (Noradrenaline)
This is the hormone that outcomes in vasoconstriction, the squeezing of the blood vessels, which allows hold or boom blood stress whilst in acute pressure.

Cortisol Hormone
Cortisol, the pressure hormone, is the maximum vital hormone withinside the frame's
reaction to pressure. Cortisol allows maintain the frame in balance, known as homeostasis, through moderating or regulating activation of the principal

anxious system, anti inflammatory and immune responses, glucose or blood sugar ranges, blood vessel and coronary heart contractions and tone, and as referenced earlier, the metabolism of fat, protein and carbohydrates.

If it's miles vital for the adrenals to provide greater cortisol in reaction to pressure, it's miles similarly vital for frame features and cortisol ranges to vary and go back to a regular kingdom after the traumatic occasion has passed. This is in part what receives reduce to rubble with Adrenal Fatigue Syndrome.

In our high-pressure culture, regularly the instances of our lives don't generate this "go back to regular" sign on that HPA axis remarks loop.

When the adrenals emerge as overworked, generating an excessive amount of cortisol, they begin to showcase symptoms and symptoms of damage and tear, not able to maintain up with the demand. When this happens, cortisol ranges drop and the frame and mind are not capable of correctly reply to traumatic or high-stress situations.

Connection to the Thyroid

The thyroid and cortisol hormones have a completely near dating. They paintings in tandem to ensure the frame has sufficient power. Hypothyroidism, wherein the thyroid doesn't produce sufficient thyroid hormone, is a completely not unusualplace condition. Prescription pills can also additionally assist repair the thyroid stability in lots of sufferers, however now no longer in all. In sufferers who do now no longer reply to this deliver of bio- same or desiccated thyroid, the signs and symptoms of mind fog, anxiety, pressure and occasional power regularly persist. The lacking hyperlink is regularly Adrenal Fatigue.

CHAPTER 2
What is Adrenal Fatigue?

Based on what you've examine so far, you'll recognize that it's a pressure condition. Adrenal Fatigue is an umbrella time period for a collection of signs and symptoms which are due to the adrenal glands now no longer operating at their optimum, and as a result, they fail to supply enough quantities of important hormones wanted with the aid of using the frame. When the adrenals prevent acting properly, all components of the frame are affected.

In healthy, low-pressure people, the remarks loop of the HPA axis works harmoniously. But, while there may be continual overproduction of cortisol and norepinephrine, the device will become desensitized, or immune, to the bad messages to "calm down". This is what finally results in continual pressure on all 3 glands and regularly consequences in some of fatigue conditions.

The overwhelming principal symptom of Adrenal Fatigue is fatigue, in particular with problem waking up withinside the morning. You can also revel in weight advantage or problem dropping weight, unexpected or abrupt weight loss, cravings for candy or salty foods, hair loss, low blood pressure, recurrent infections and sluggish healing.

We'll get into extra element approximately the symptoms and symptoms and signs and symptoms of Adrenal Fatigue in Chapter 4.

What Causes Adrenal Fatigue?

Western society is an increasing number of speedy-paced, and it's far clearly extra tough than it was, even 50 years ago, to take a spoil and relaxation. Not simply bodily, however emotionally and mentally. Things like technology, wherein our gadgets observe a lot of us to bed, profession pressures, dating and own circle of relatives issues, can all upload as much as generate a steady flow of pressure. At a sure factor a lot of us prevent being capable of accurately reply while heightened or extreme pressure activities occur, and now and again this results in an incapability to manage or characteristic with the stresses of daily living.

Boiled right all the way down to basics, pressure reasons Adrenal Fatigue. Your adrenal glands

clearly grow to be much less and much less capable of address the hormone-manufacturing needs pressure is putting on them.

What reasons Adrenal Fatigue in a single man or woman can be pretty distinct from the motive in another. Pinpointing the precise motive may be tough. The symptoms and symptoms and signs and symptoms increase slowly, now and again over a decade or extra. It isn't always unusual for a person to go through Adrenal Fatigue Syndrome and in no way honestly recognize precisely what the cause was. There are some of reasons that may be grouped into six principal categories, in no precise order:

#1: Trauma
A single, bodily demanding occasion can result in Adrenal Fatigue, which

now and again manifests years later. Car accidents, principal surgery, extreme sports activities accidents or different activities all fall into this category.

#2: Chronic Disease
Coping with continual infection or ailment locations above-regular needs in your adrenal glands. Fibromyalgia, continual pain, Lyme ailment, asthma, diabetes or arthritis can also additionally all be factors.

#3: Not Enough Sleep
Most latest surveys endorse Americans are becoming a median of simply over 6 hours of sleep in step with night time. That's down from a median of eight hours of sleep each night time 50 to a hundred years ago, and brief of the eight – nine hours of relaxation the professionals endorse we want earlier than we're prone to growing sleep issues and different associated illnesses.

#4: Emotional Stress
Different from the pressure due to bodily trauma, emotional pressure can also additionally sense plausible withinside the brief time period. However, prolonged durations beneathneath emotional pressure can motive, or at the least make a contribution to, Adrenal Fatigue. Whether it's a terrible boss at paintings, an sad dating, having a ill child, moving, or the demise of a own circle of relatives member, emotional pressure can grow to be continual if the underlying motive isn't dealt with.

#5: Poor Diet, Crash Dieting & Addictions
You've heard the saying 'you're what you eat'. Unhealthy ingesting patterns that consist of an excessive amount of speedy food, excessive delicate sugar and fats intake, and yo-yo or crash weight-reduction plan all positioned a extraordinary stress at the adrenal glands as they conflict to hold homeostasis withinside the frame. Addictions to alcohol, pills, and ingesting issues will all motive your adrenals to paintings tougher and will increase the hazard they'll grow to be fatigued.

#6: Pollutants and Chemicals (Addictions)
'Toxic load' is a word used to explain the general degree of toxicity in our environments. Air pollutants (from cars, industry), antibiotics in meat, insecticides on culmination and vegetables, even chlorine in our consuming water. All of those, and greater, are chemical compounds that could have a fabric and bad effect on our average health, together with the adrenals. Some

of those chemical compounds in reality disrupt adrenal characteristic, forcing the opposite elements of the HPA axis to modify and fill the void.

Four Levels of Adrenal Fatigue

All Adrenal Fatigue isn't the identical and signs can range significantly among individuals. In a unmarried person the kind and diploma of signs can extrade over time. What I've learned, though, is that there are commonly 4 exceptional stages of Adrenal Fatigue, and those stages constitute the improvement technique of adrenal exhaustion.

Level One: Initial Stress Response

This is the primary section of strain response, at some point of which the frame continues to be making sufficient of the hormones had to effectively reply to a strain trigger. Blood assessments administered whilst on this degree could display better stages of cortisol, adrenaline, norepinephrine, insulin and DHEA.

It's everyday for us to slide inside and outside of degree one numerous instances at some point of our lives, and whilst sleep may also start to suffer, signs are not often bothersome sufficient to file or are looking for treatment.

Level Two: Alarm

Alarm bells begin to ring because the endocrine machine begins offevolved to divert sources from intercourse hormone manufacturing over to strain hormone manufacturing. In degree there is usually a chronic feeling of being worn-out however hyper-alert: sunlight hours alertness to characteristic generally with a fatigue crash withinside the evening. Unhealthy

dependence on caffeine or alcohol and different materials regularly develops withinside the alarm stage.

Level Three: Resistance

The frame demonstrates its brilliance in degree , adapting to extended strain via way of means of generating greater strain hormones and less intercourse hormones.
Testosterone and DHEA stages drop in order that the endocrine machine can hold generating greater cortisol. Life and task characteristic regularly nevertheless seem everyday whilst in degree three, however major signs together with reduced intercourse drive, ordinary infections and tiredness begin to take their toll.
A man or woman can loaf around in 'resistance' territory for months, and

occasionally even years.

Level Four: Burnout

All the sources used to divert hormone manufacturing to cortisol manufacturing are used up, or even cortisol stages start to drop. Low intercourse hormones, low strain hormones, and occasional neurotransmitters too. It's the crash that regularly arrives after lengthy intervals of huge strain. Here the signs may be referred to in the course of the frame: excessive fatigue, apathy, depression, anxiety, weight loss, and depression, to call only a few. In burnout, you'll regularly locate which you can't hold up with the every day tempo that has been "everyday" to your existence to this point. Recovery from burnout regularly calls for a complete way of life extrade, together with wholesome doses of each persistence and time.

CHAPTER 3
Overlooked, Misdiagnosed, Misunderstood

Adrenal Fatigue is particularly controversial. The clinical network is cut up as to whether or not there's a systematic foundation for a analysis of Adrenal Fatigue, and plenty of argue there can be different scientifically tested diagnoses to give an explanation for Adrenal Fatigue signs.

It's proper there are some of different ailments that may be related to Adrenal Fatigue: fibromyalgia, persistent fatigue syndrome, hypothyroidism, estrogen dominance, ovarian-adrenal-thyroid imbalance syndrome, and others. Generalized signs can regularly overlap. Proponents of Adrenal Fatigue trust that during a few instances AFS is the underlying motive of those different conditions. Allow me to attempt to paint a clean image of why I trust this clinical struggle exists.

Adrenal Insufficiency Versus Adrenal Fatigue

Adrenal insufficiency, referred to as Addison's Disease, stocks most of the signs of Adrenal Fatigue, however they're plenty greater extreme. Addison's is regularly additionally observed via way of means of extended vomiting, extreme muscle weakness, very low blood strain or maybe shock, profound sleepiness or maybe coma. If you watched this sounds serious, you're sincerely correct. A man or woman with those signs can be in adrenal disaster and desires emergency clinical treatment.

Adrenal insufficiency happens while the adrenal glands are not able to function, if they're absent or were eliminated. Most frequently adrenal insufficiency is the end result of an autoimmune disorder, in which the body's very own immune machine assaults the cells of the adrenal glands. Infection, which includes tuberculosis, also can be a cause. And in instances in which the adrenal glands were surgically eliminated there may be apparent number one adrenal insufficiency.

Taking artificial steroid medicinal drugs like prednisolone, prednisone and dexamethasone also can bring about adrenal insufficiency as it hints the pituitary gland into questioning there may be greater than sufficient cortisol withinside the bloodstream, so it doesn't inform the adrenals to fabricate any greater.

Endocrinologists warn that through taking adrenal dietary supplements containing extracts of lively adrenal hormone unnecessarily may also render the adrenal glands vain and they will now no longer paintings while they're wished most. Many critical ailments, like rheumatic diseases, cancer, hepatitis C and greater, proportion signs which includes fatigue, and self-medicating with those adrenal dietary supplements may also permit the underlying disorder to development undetected for too lengthy earlier than detection.

History of Adrenal Fatigue

Once Dr. Thomas Addison first offered his concept on a disorder of the "suprarenal capsules" (nowadays known as adrenal glands) that offered as an anemia-like situation withinside the mid-1800s. Subsequently it have become referred to as Addison's Disease. Addison's findings induced similarly studies and brought about what have become the sphere of endocrinology.

Later that century, physicians commenced the usage of extracts from porcine adrenal cells (yup, pigs) to deal with each Addison's Disease and the milder situation known as hypoadrenia.

"Adrenal Fatigue" as a time period commenced rising withinside the past due 1990's. That's while Dr. James L. Wilson, a naturopath and chiropractor with 3 PhD's, commenced the usage of it to explain a set of signs that have been comparable throughout some of tired, immune-compromised patients.

The debate among one-of-a-kind factions of the clinical network over the life of Adrenal Fatigue has now no longer modified a good deal withinside the ultimate century.

What's on the center of this debate? The query of whether or not the road among fitness and infection is as strong as black and white, in which a affected person is both ill or healthy, or whether or not there may be complete spectrum on which there are numerous levels among severely unwell and absolutely healthy.

Illness-Wellness Continuum

In 1972, John W. Travis first proposed the idea of the "infection-wellness" continuum. Travis, founding father of The Wellness Resource Centre in Mill Valley, California, opined that it have to take drastically greater than the easy absence of detectable 'infection' to decide whether or not a person was "well".

On the some distance left of Travis' continuum is early or pre-mature death. In the

center is a impartial factor in which there may be no proof of both infection or wellness. On the some distance proper of the continuum is a excessive degree of wellness. And in among the 2 points, from left to proper, are:

- Disability
- Symptoms
- Signs
- Neutral (no detectible illness or wellness)
- Awareness
- Education
- Growth

This continuum, which through the manner echoes the view of the World Health Organization, contradicts the techniques of fitness experts that best engage, diagnose and deal with people while they may be absolutely ill, at the left- hand aspect of the continuum: that is, displaying signs, signs or even incapacity associated with disorder.

Travis additionally believes that the "attitude" of every person performs a great function in in which they fall at the continuum. Those with a nice outlook on existence can have higher fitness consequences than people with a bad outlook on existence, irrespective of the presence or absence of laboratory-showed disorder.

Subclinical Versus Clinical

There are many ailments that stay under the brink of medical laboratory detection: examples encompass rheumatoid arthritis, moderate hypothyroidism and diabetes. Adrenal Fatigue is the subclinical syndrome of Adrenal Insufficiency, or Addison's disorder. By the time the laboratory exams "prove" adrenal insufficiency, frequently the best remedy choice is lifelong alternative of bio-same corticosteroids.

Diagnostic techniques and laboratory exams are especially mechanized and do now no longer consider the great strong point of every person's body. No special history, no examine nutrition, way of life or genetic elements thru which to view lab check results.

Reliance on laboratory take a look at outcomes which might be skewed to an all or not anything technique go away no room to remember Adrenal Fatigue Syndrome as subclinical to Addison's Disease, or that moderate versions of outcomes inside a "normal"
variety may also certainly be signs of terrible adrenal fitness in a few sufferers. Doctors carrying those all or not anything blinders condemn sufferers such as you and me to both go through needlessly or seek on our very own for solutions.

Advances in preventive and so-known as opportunity medication are supporting the ones sufferers. In many instances they're capable of forestall ailment improvement while it's miles nevertheless in this "sub-clinical" kingdom in order that it does now no longer end up greater serious.

Large Patient Pool

There is a developing swell of people such as you who're inclined and geared up to take their fitness into their very own fingers and search for approaches to assist themselves to heal and sense better. According to Dr. Michael Lam (a Medical Doctor with a Masters of Public Health and certification from the American Board of Anti- Aging Medicine who makes a speciality of Adrenal Fatigue and dietary medication), over 50 percentage of the person populace will be afflicted by Adrenal Fatigue in some unspecified time in the future of their lifetime.

At the time of this writing, 1.forty five million seek outcomes had been again after entering "Adrenal Fatigue" into Google's seek engine. That's a whole lot of hobby and hobby for a syndrome that conventional medication doesn't with no trouble apprehend.

There is presently no easy laboratory take a look at that may be perceive or affirm a prognosis of Adrenal Fatigue. This is, as a minimum in part, what's at the foundation of the controversy, or conflict, among scientific and fitness practitioners over Adrenal Fatigue (and different situations).

In many sufferers, laboratory blood assessments will flip up "normal", leaving the affected person to sense like she or he is "crazy", imagining things, or a hypochondriac. Don't melancholy if that is happening, or has happened, to you! Keep reading. I can assist.

Medical Evolution

Let's recollect that till very recently, the Western medication network additionally didn't apprehend persistent fatigue syndrome, fibromyalgia, chiropractors, naturopaths or Chinese medication, which has been practiced for lots of years. We best must appearance again a hundred years or so that you could discover that "hysteria" turned into a catchall description for a bunch of "female" troubles from

fainting to anxiety, sleeplessness to irritability and nervousness, with questionable strategies of treatment. Can it's one of these stretch to suppose that medication will capture up and Adrenal Fatigue turns into a greater broadly diagnosed syndrome?

As an increasing number of people take our severa bodily court cases to our scientific doctors, who inform us "your assessments are all negative", after which retain to do our very own studies and take our fitness into our very own fingers, the scientific network can have an increasing number of motives to regulate their technique.

CHAPTER 4
Adrenal Fatigue. Do You Have It?

As I simply referenced in Chapter 3, different scientific situations can produce the identical signs and symptoms as Adrenal Fatigue. It is critical to make certain you've got got identified, and been handled for, every other situations or fitness elements that can be contributing for your signs and symptoms earlier than achieving a prognosis of Adrenal Fatigue.

Adrenal Fatigue Syndrome affords with a aggregate of signs and symptoms that together, along side the absence of every other formal scientific prognosis, brings you to the belief that your adrenal glands are under-functioning, or fatigued.

Signs and Symptoms of Adrenal Fatigue

There are not unusualplace symptoms and symptoms and signs and symptoms, skilled with the aid of using almost every person with Adrenal Fatigue in various tiers or intensity. These are:

- Fatigue
- Weight gain tendency, especially around the waist
- Frequent flu or other respiratory diseases or infections that last longer than normal
- Low sex drive
- Dizziness or lightheadedness when standing
- Poor memory and muddled thinking
- Low morning energy, as well as in the late afternoon
- Need caffeine or other stimulants to start the day
- Meals bring temporary relief
- Food cravings for fatty, salty and sugary foods
- Unexplained neck, upper or lower back pain
- Increased PMS, with periods that are heavy and stop, or almost stop, on about day 4, starting again on day 5 or 6
- Startle easily
- Feeling overwhelmed, trouble managing stress and responsibility
- Body temperature issues: cold hands and feet, warm face, hot flashes
- Unexplained hair loss, and
- Multiple allergies or sensitivities to food

Physical Signs

Fatigue

Fatigue is the most important symptom of Adrenal Fatigue, and is gift to a few diploma in each affected person with AFS. In particular, upon waking withinside the morning, no matter how lengthy or how excellent a nap you've had, feeling gradual and simply now no longer capable of "wake up" withinside the morning is a key symptom.

- Puffy, swollen eyes in the morning,
- Battling fatigue throughout the day, with a significant low in the late afternoon
- Disrupted sleep, and

- Feeling the most energetic in the evening

Weight Gain or Changes, Food Cravings

- Abdominal fat accumulation that is unexplained
- Need for coffee or other stimulants to "get going" in the morning
- Cravings for fatty foods, and
- Cravings for salty or sweet foods

Blood Pressure

- Consistent low blood pressure, and
- Dizziness while getting up from mendacity or sitting

Anxiety

- Inability to relax, despite fatigue, feeling wired Feelings of
- low self-esteem and depression Panic attacks, and
- Feeling of adrenalin rushes

Hormones/Libido

- Low thyroid function (hypothyroidism) that doesn't seem to respond to medication, and
- Low sex drive

Female Issues

- Post partum fatigue and depression
- Recurrent miscarriages, specifically for the duration of 1st trimester Painful
- menstrual cramps or unexplained overlooked intervals Irregular menstrual
- cycle
- Ovarian cysts Uterine fibroids
- Endometriosis, and
- Premature menopause

Frequent Infections, Slow Healing
Examples include:

- Recurring urinary tract infections (UTI)
- Unexplained eye infections, and/or
- Slower than normal healing of even minor cuts and bruises

Mental or Emotional Signs

- Fuzzy thinking, brain fog or chronic racing thoughts
- Irritability, especially under stress
- Coping ability and emotions
- Can't focus or concentrate
- Feeling unable to cope with stress
- Mild depression, and
- Feeling frazzled or scatter-brained

Miscellaneous Signs

- Hair loss
- Temperature intolerance (sensitivity to heat and sunlight, cold hands and feet)
- Dry or prematurely aging skin
- Chronic tinnitus (ringing in the ear)
- Dark circles under the eyes that don't disappear with rest
- Body aches and joint pain, and
- Muscle weakness, loss of muscle mass

Testing (or Lack There of)

Given the rift withinside the scientific network over whether or not certainly

Adrenal Fatigue exists, I suggest you to take first rate care as you figure to decide whether or not you certainly may also be afflicted by the syndrome.

Consult your physician, however be organized for her or him to inform you not anything is incorrect. Listen in your instinct. If you KNOW some thing is certainly incorrect with you, be prepared now no longer to permit your physician's lack of ability to assist get you down.

So, go to your physician, provide an explanation for your signs, and ask for a popular checkup and a complete blood take a look at to make certain you don't produce other underlying nutrient deficiencies (which includes low nutrition B12, iron or nutrition D, to call only a few), hormonal imbalances or different fitness situations that want to be addressed.

If, after complete exams were completed, different reasons have both been dominated out or addressed, and you continue to have the identical signs, then you can take into account the motive of your signs to be Adrenal Fatigue.

Unfortunately, your physician or might not be inclined to refer you to all the endorsed exams stated underneath due to the fact they're regularly now no longer blanketed through insurance. If that is the case, you can additionally paintings with an opportunity fitness care practitioner with revel in in Adrenal Fatigue (if possible, as they will be tough to find). Discuss all of your symptoms and symptoms and signs with them, what different scientific situations were diagnosed and/or dealt with through your physician, and ask for a saliva take a look at.

Ask to peer the real lab effects, after which use the facts underneath that will help you interpret the findings and stability that towards what your physician or practitioner is telling you.

Cortisol Tests
Cortisol may be measured through urine, blood or saliva, and every physician may have his or her preference. Many take into account saliva the maximum correct method, because it suggests cortisol stages at a cell level.

A unmarried cortiSol take a look at isn't always enough. Cortisol commonly spikes withinside the morning, losing off over the route of the day. So, as a way to properly decide the characteristic of your adrenal glands in generating cortisol, measurements taken at some of factors at some stage in the day and mapped over a 24 hour length will inform your physician lots extra than a unmarried take a look at.

If you're seeing a health practitioner who doesn't have education or revel in, or doesn't consider in Adrenal Fatigue, then the effects are possibly now no longer going to be as it should be interpreted. The laboratory's reference levels are regularly so massive that most effective the maximum severe effects – at both the excessive or low end – could be flagged.

What are those "ordinary" levels? They will range from laboratory to laboratory, and your physician, if he/she is reasonably progressive, may also make modifications to what he/she considers ordinary primarily based totally for your fitness and different factors.

As a popular manual morning cortisol of 5 – 23 micrograms in step with deciliter (mcg/dL) withinside the morning or among 3 – sixteen mcg/dL withinside the afternoon might be considered "ordinary". The mission is that even though effects fall inside this "ordinary" range, this can now no longer truly rule out Adrenal Fatigue. It can be extra useful to appearance at "top-quality" levels, alternatively than "ordinary", or to take your effects to an opportunity remedy practitioner with understanding in Adrenal Fatigue.

ACTH
Once your baseline cortisol stages were mapped, an ACTH (adrenal corticotrophin hormone) mission take a look at can be useful.

You could be injected with an ACTH dose, which mimics strain in stimulating your adrenal hormone production. Your cortisol stages might be examined again. As lengthy as there's a marked spike, displaying as about doubled for your blood take a look at in comparison to the baseline cortisol take a look at, your adrenals are possibly functioning well. If the cortisol spike is much less than double, it indicates underperforming adrenals.

Thyroid
The thyroid additionally works on a remarks loop with the hypothalamus and pituitary glands, and this courting is referred to as the HPT axis. Remember that the adrenal glands are part of the HPA axis, and top-quality characteristic is interrelated. They're all a part of the endocrine system. Any weakening of the pituitary or hypothalamus glands, which takes place in Adrenal Fatigue, can bring about decrease thyroid characteristic. The mission is that the usual levels for "ordinary" utilized by labs and the medical doctors who interpret the exams don't properly take into account the nuances of hypothyroidism, nor the truth that hypothyroidism itself can be because of Adrenal Fatigue.

TSH
The pituitary gland produces thyroid-stimulating hormone (TSH), which in

flip activates the thyroid to generate T3 and T4. If your thyroid gland is thankfully churning out ok quantities of T3 and T4, your TSH stages could be decrease due to the fact the thyroid doesn't want as lots stimulation. On the opposite hand, in case your T3 and T4 stages are decrease, indicating you're hypothyroid, then your TSH will in all likelihood be higher, due to the fact your hypothalamus is sending greater thyroid stimulating hormone, telling your thyroid it wishes to supply greater of the important T3 and T4 hormones.

The laboratory reference levels for "regular" TSH range barely lab to lab, however commonly fall withinside the zero.4 – 4.zero gadgets in line with milliliter variety. Those affected by Adrenal Fatigue frequently have poorly acting thyroid glands and the TSH stage could be above 2.zero. Perhaps now no longer sufficient to spark off your clinical medical doctor to reserve treatment, however, blended with different assessments, may also assist you and your opportunity medication expert to attain a prognosis of Adrenal Fatigue.

T3 and T4

T4 is greater plentiful withinside the bloodstream, however T3 is virtually accountable for maximum of the body's metabolic activity. Both T3 and T4 are made from loose, or "unbound", hormones which can be to be had to your tissues and cells to apply proper away, at the side of hormone that is "bound" to protein cells. The Free T3 and T4 is the maximum beneficial dimension because it offers a clearer image to diagnosticians. For overall T4, the regular variety for adults is ready five to fourteen mcg/dL (micrograms in line with deciliter), even as loose T4's regular variety is ready zero.8 – two hundred ng/dL (nanograms in line with deciliter). For overall T3, search for outcomes among approximately eighty and two hundred ng/dL and 2.3 – 4.2 pg/dL (pictograms in line with deciliter) without spending a dime T3.

Side Note: If you observed you've got got a thyroid hassle However the above thyroid assessments are within "regular" lab levels in keeping with your medical doctor, don't forget having a complete thyroid panel check completed, which incorporates TSH, Free T4, Free T3, Reverse T3, and Thyroid Antibodies. However, all of those assessments are frequently NOT executed through docs as they will depend upon TSH alone, which does now no longer offer a complete review of thyroid function. You may also pick to go to a innovative thyroid professional or opportunity healthcare practitioner instead. Iodine deficiency also can motive adrenal and thyroid symptoms. If you observed you've got got iodine deficiency, paintings with a expert to behavior checking out and administer iodine supplementation (that is a sensitive procedure that calls for tailor-made steering from a knowledgeable, iodine-conscious practitioner).

Blood Pressure Test

Comparing outcomes of blood stress assessments among sitting and status positions can monitor capability Adrenal Fatigue. The first studying must be taken after you've been resting for approximately five mins and are pretty relaxed. Then get up proper away, and take your blood stress again.

Increased Pressure and Heart Rate

Your blood stress must growth whilst you get up that allows you to preserve blood flowing in your brain. A ten to 20 factor growth, at the side of multiplied coronary heart rate, suggests wholesome adrenal function.

Static Rates Between Sitting and Standing

If you're very athletic, there can be little or no alternate in blood stress among the resting and status positions. In this case, no alternate in stress might imply regular adrenal function.

Drop in Blood Pressure

If your adrenals are not able to supply sufficient adrenaline and cortisol, while you are taking your 2d dimension upon status you'll note a drop in blood stress and you could sense dizzy.

Saliva Test

Saliva assessments are gaining credibility and reputation through clinical docs as dependable determinants of cortisol stages. Your medical doctor or opportunity clinical

practitioner can order the saliva check, and that is the satisfactory solution.

Because your adrenal glands control all your strain responses, checking cortisol stages at various instances of the day are important to show fluctuations withinside the strain reaction that can be abnormal.

The check entails gathering saliva at 4 distinctive factors for the duration of the day (i.e. 8am, noon, 4pm and simply earlier than midnight) after which measuring the cortisol, estrogen, progesterone, DHEAS and testosterone stages.

Self Diagnosing

If you aren't capable of discover a right healthcare practitioner to paintings with, otherwise you truely can't come up with the money for one (a few coverage plans do now no longer appropriately cowl opportunity fitness experts or their referred testing), then right here is a few extra data that will help you self-diagnose. Adrenal Fatigue is one of the few scientific situations that may be self-recognized and self treated. I did it, and I am feeling an entire lot better.

Home Saliva Tests
There are a developing range of Internet reassets that allows you to order your very own saliva "home-check" to test your cortisol profile, and maximum of those laboratories are right and reliable. Just watch out for web sites in an effort to additionally attempt to promote you vitamins, herbs or supplements. In different words, the unfairness will exist to attempt to expose which you require the goods they're selling.

Pupillary Response Test
Physicians like Dr. Jeffrey Dach, Dr. Lawrence Wilson and Dr. James L. Wilson all communicate approximately a pupillary reaction check you may do at home. This check can assist screen early ranges of Adrenal Fatigue, however need to now no longer be taken in isolation as some of different situations can have an effect on the effects of this kind of check. Pupillary reaction check isn't always as crucial in diagnosing Adrenal Fatigue as blood sugar manage or blood strain renovation tests.

How to Do the Test
You want a vulnerable flashlight, or penlight, a darkish room, a mirror, and a stopwatch (you may use an app to your smartphone).

1. Go into the darkish room, and live withinside the darkish for some minutes

   to allow your eyes regulate to the darkish.
2. Standing in the front of the mirror, preserve the mild to the aspect of your head and shine the mild from the aspect throughout one eye, now no longer at once into it.
3. Keep the mild shining gradually throughout the attention and watch your scholar. You need to word that it contracts right now while the mild hits it.
4. Time how lengthy your scholar holds the contraction earlier than it dilates, which it'll... after which it'll settlement again.

What it Means
The duration of time your scholar holds the contraction earlier than it dilates,

and whether or not it "bounces" round dilating/contracting below the mild, may be a trademark of Adrenal Fatigue.

The longer your scholar can preserve the contraction, the better. If your scholar can preserve contraction for 30 or extra seconds earlier than it dilates again, that's a extraordinary signal which you aren't in early ranges of Adrenal Fatigue.

Pulsing is likewise adequate as it indicates your frame is adjusting. Where there are issues are while your scholar does now no longer settlement at all.

CHAPTER 5
Curing Adrenal Fatigue Naturally: Diet, Vitamins & Supplements

When you're below pressure, your frame wishes extra nutritious gasoline than it might otherwise. The key right here is nutritious. Fast meals simply ain't it. Along with what you consume, *whilst you consume is likewise crucial.* Eating often – and ingesting enough
– allows maintain cortisol degrees solid so the adrenal glands don't ought to paintings pretty so hard. The answer is to take withinside the proper gasoline and decrease capability nutritional stressors to make certain our our bodies run easily and optimally, which as a result, will useful resource in recovery Adrenal Fatigue.

Based by myself private recovery revel in with Adrenal Fatigue, plus many achievement tales of actual people, I actually have ad infinitum researched the consequences of weight-reduction plan in recovery the human frame – and the answer appears so simple. In curing Adrenal Fatigue, selected a weight-reduction plan this is simple, entire, and springs from nature; inclusive of plant-primarily based totally, excessive nutrient entire meals. Eating a weight-reduction plan wealthy in plant-primarily based totally meals is established to lower the general hazard of disorder and locations much less pressure on our adrenal glands, which I will cope with in extra element at some point of this chapter.

Though this could now no longer be famend as a 'conventional' technique in a society complete of marketing, fad diets and falsity, there are numerous educated, distinctly trained, and properly-reputable scientific docs who percentage this view (and from whom I actually have learned), who've efficaciously helped their sufferers end up properly again. You may locate different opposing techniques obtainable that declare to treatment Adrenal Fatigue, to which I disagree – I actually have attempted those hints and discovered they made my signs and symptoms worse and did now no longer paintings for me withinside the lengthy-term.

Dr. Neal Barnard has written notably approximately stopping most cancers with a plant-primarily based totally weight-reduction plan. He references facts that indicates the hazard of demise from most cancers will increase among 14 and 50 percentage for individuals who often consume pink and processed meats and who eat excessive-fats dairy. Dr. Dean Ornish, Dr. John McDougall, Dr. Joel Fuhrman and Dr. Caldwell Esselstyn are additionally

Proactive nutrients experts, every selling a eating regimen this is plant-primarily based totally and occasional in fats to prevent, or reverse, coronary heart ailment and different illnesses. If you do your very own research, as I have, you'll discover different examples of scientific medical doctors who have 'visible the light' and are selling the electricity of desire in eating regimen and way of life in reversing or stopping ailment and dramatically enhancing how we experience. Adrenal Fatigue is one of the syndromes that may be reversed with a touch schooling and effort, and it's my delight that will help you alongside your journey.

Diet

Choose the Right Foods

Plant-Based Foods
A plant-primarily based totally eating regimen is focused on vegetables, end result, complete grains (ideally gluten unfastened sorts for adrenal recuperation), legumes, nuts and seeds, with very little animal products. Some examples may also consist of cucumbers, apples, leafy greens, broccoli, mushrooms, brown rice, berries, beans, lentils and peas, simply to call a few. Colorful plant meals comprise herbal phytochemicals, fiber and antioxidants (which assist defend our our bodies from ailment and helps our basic health), and gives our our bodies with ample vitamins which includes iron and calcium. Though consuming one hundred percentage plant-primarily based totally is optimal, in case you are transitioning, I do inspire you try and have as a minimum eighty five percentage of your eating regimen (the extra the higher) made up of those nutrient-dense, non-processed meals for quicker healing. You will be aware how tons higher you begin to experience very quickly.

Whole Foods

The contrary of processed. It certainly approach taking note of consuming meals that appears as near what it did whilst it changed into developing in nature, with the least quantity of processing possible. Not that each one processing is bad, either. The processing you do on your very own kitchen, say making applesauce from herbal apples, is great and needn't be avoided. Ready-made meals or condiments that comprise easy, natural, plant-primarily based totally substances also are a great addition for your complete meals meals – you'll discover ways to examine labels like a pro.

The Carb Conundrum

Carbohydrates are the macronutrient our our bodies require withinside the largest

quantities, as they may be our essential supply of strength and gas for our our bodies (and our minds!) to characteristic optimally – an critical key in preventing low moods and strength stages in Adrenal Fatigue.

Many processed carbohydrate meals are considered 'easy carbs', which could metabolize speedy and become short bursts of strength highs and lows. Examples of processed easy carbs comprise white desk sugar, discovered in jams and jellies, gentle liquids or candies, which comprise little dietary benefit.

Avoid those processed carbs and choose complete meals containing herbal, easy sugars (like fruit), which might be higher metabolized with the aid of using the frame with its fiber, proteins, nutrients and minerals nevertheless in tact.

Many humans worry fruit beneathneath the guise that it's miles the only offender for blood sugar spikes. This, however, is inaccurate and relies upon how the sugars are harmonized with extra fat withinside the eating regimen (specifically saturated fats), which I will deal with withinside the following section. During the preliminary degrees of your recuperation whilst your frame is adjusting to its new eating regimen, it's exceptional to eat end result and sparkling juices in advance withinside the day, and as your Adrenal Fatigue stabilizes you can preserve to include extra end result into your eating regimen to revel in in abundance.

'Complex carbs' also are complete of fiber, nutrients and minerals. They are enjoyable as they take longer to digest, are used by the frame for long-time period strength release, and might truely accelerate your metabolism in order that your frame burns energy extra efficiently. Examples consist of complete plant meals like starchy vegetables (potatoes, candy potatoes, yams, pumpkin and corn), and complete grains (ideally gluten unfastened) – choose brown rice over white rice, specially in the course of the primary segment of healing. These are all exquisite alternatives to consist of on your eating regimen at any time of day.

Don't Avoid Carbs

It's regarding to peer such a lot of women and men reduce carbohydrates out in their eating regimen withinside the hopes they may lose weight, while in reality, it may have pretty the other bring about the long-time period. Avoiding carbs is a not unusualplace mistake and might make Adrenal Fatigue worse, and here's why.

We've pointed out the relationship among hypothyroidism and Adrenal Fatigue. Carbs without delay have an effect on thyroid characteristic. Carbohydrates get transformed into the glucose (sugar), which matches collectively with insulin to offer strength.

Insulin is wanted to transform T4 (the inactive hormone) into T3 (the energetic hormone). Low carbs = low insulin = low thyroid and accelerated symptoms, along with long-time period weight gain.

Cortisol, the primary hormone produced via way of means of the adrenal glands, has a tendency to boom whilst on a low carb weight-reduction plan due to the fact the frame desires to stability out its glucose ranges. This approach it's far a ability stressor on your adrenal system. If you're already affected by Adrenal Fatigue Syndrome, or are prone and suspect you could have AFS, including a low carb weight-reduction plan to a traumatic job, terrible sleep and perhaps immoderate exercise, and voila. You've simply perfected the recipe for burnout!

Excess fats withinside the blood (specifically from animal merchandise and processed oils) obstructs the shipping of glucose to our cells for electricity, which overworks our adrenals, creates an adrenalin rush, and effects in a blood sugar spike or insulin resistance. Some human beings want to deal with this hassle via way of means of getting rid of carbohydrates from their weight-reduction plan. You may want to expect this could make sense, right? But this indicates maximum in their weight-reduction plan could be made from fat and protein
– and as we realize via way of means of now, an entire host of fitness issues can appear if the frame is missing an important supply of gas to feature properly.

Maintaining Solid glucose ranges will offer you with most fulfilling fats burning efficiency, lengthen your electricity ranges, have a fantastic impact in your temper and manage your urge for food while minimizing meals cravings. So, don't be scared of complicated carbohydrates and herbal sugars in plant-primarily based totally complete ingredients.

Limit Gluten Grains and Concentrated Sugar

These culprits may also make contributions to impaired insulin response, HPA disorder and popular inflammation. Lara Briden, a Canadian-educated Naturopathic Doctor now certified and practising in Australia, calls gluten grains and focused sugar "un-mild carbs", and promotes avoidance for people with hormone imbalance problems like Adrenal Fatigue.

But Briden and different specialists do suggest intake of "mild carbs", which might be the carbs that don't sell inflammation. Root greens like beet, potato and candy potato, and complete grains like brown rice, quinoa, buckwheat, millet or amaranth are tremendous complicated carbohydrates to feed an adrenal fatigued frame. Eating slight quantities is suggested as helpful in assisting adrenal feature.

It is likewise very essential to become aware of and dispose of another ingredients which you are allergic or illiberal to. Food sensitivities are very not unsualplace and can be worsening your symptoms. Common offenders encompass wheat, gluten, dairy, eggs, soy and plenty of others.

What About Protein?

Proteins are discovered in all ingredients (even in culmination and greens) in enough quantities for our our bodies to thrive. For the preliminary remedy of Adrenal Fatigue though, it's far advocated to often devour a small part of protein wealthy meals (plant-primarily based totally, of course, like beans, nuts, seeds, or legumes) together with your mild, gradual carbs. This will bring about even higher blood sugar stability – powerful for the ones folks with insulin sensitivities, which is available in hand with having Adrenal Fatigue. If you pick out to devour soy merchandise (pleasant carefully in case you aren't illiberal or sensitive), choose natural soy with the least processing possible, inclusive of tempeh or natural tofu.

There are various critiques concerning day by day macronutrient ratios – what labored for me throughout my recovery system turned into a degree of about 60% carbohydrates, 25% protein and 15% fats. Rather than being meticulous with this, I suggest which you honestly make sure fats does now no longer exceed about 20 to 25% of your day by day intake, and make certain you're ingesting extra proper carbohydrates than proteins to preserve enough electricity ranges. Everyone's protocol may be barely different, as every person's metabolic price and nation of fitness is different. The universal emphasis is on complete ingredients, so that you may also test a touch with ratios to sense what works satisfactory to your frame and what is going to satisfactory allow you to paste to an entire ingredients weight-reduction plan. As your frame adjusts to its new weight-reduction plan, starts to heal and balances its insulin, you could slowly boom your carbohydrate ratio to in which you sense maximum satisfied.

Facts About Fat

Fats are an critical a part of our weight loss program, however it's far the first-class and amount of fats that we ought to be aware of. We regularly pay attention approximately the advantages of a Mediterranean weight loss program and prefer to characteristic this to using olive oil, however what's regularly neglected is the overall nutritional pattern – a menu wealthy in unrefined plant ingredients with a totally restricted consumption of dairy and meat.

What has labored efficiently for lots human beings who've suffered from Adrenal Fatigue is getting rid of saturated fat (usually located in animal products) and restricting processed oils, but nonetheless taking part in the complete meals model moderately to get hold of complete dietary benefit (i.e. complete olives in place of olive oil, coconut meat in place of coconut oil, avocado over avocado oil, complete nuts and seeds over nut oils).

According to Dr. John McDougall, *"our our bodies can synthesize maximum fat from carbohydrates and there are only some unsaturated fat that our our bodies can't make through themselves"*. As a result, there's no want to overload our our bodies with extra fat and processed oils, that may overwork our pancreas and forces our adrenal glands to provide extra adrenaline (which over time, can bring about a large number of fitness issues as a result of negative weight loss program, which includes Adrenal Fatigue).

Contrary to various opinions, processed oils, which includes vegetable oils, olive or maybe coconut oil, aren't wholesome especially for the ones affected by Adrenal Fatigue. Hydrogenated oils, despite the fact that they sound like they arrive from a wholesome source, like soybean, corn or canola, have a tendency to be very inflammatory and might stimulate your adrenal glands – and while heated grow to be rancid and carcinogenic. Oils also are calorie dense while thinking about their low nutrient value, as they're stripped of fiber, making them effortlessly absorbed into the bloodstream – a recipe for clean fats storage.

Minimizing oils can be a project at first, so strive cooking with vegetable broths, natural soy sauce (tamari), tomato juice or a sprint of water while sautéing in a non-stick frying pan. In baking, you may update oil with ingredients like applesauce or mashed bananas to feature texture and moisture.

Calorie Restriction? Never.
Unfortunately, our preference for fast and rapid effects can regularly negatively have an effect on our fitness. Crash diets and calorie limit may get you for your aim weight 'faster' withinside the short-term, however ask yourself, will you be able to sustain the same dietary habits forever? Will you keep the weight off? And will this harm your health and your metabolism in the long-term? You *WILL* be able to get to a healthy weight and maintain it once you have healed your body and consistently eat healthfully. Patience and consistency is key.

It's sincerely critical now no longer to beneathneath devour. Not consuming sufficient or going long

intervals with out a nutritious snack can placed your frame into extra stress. It thinks there can be hunger at the horizon and is going into safety mode (read*: stress)*, placing extra needs to your already-worn-out adrenals. Don't starve your cells of herbal electricity through heading off or significantly proscribing meals – make certain to hold your frame fuelled in the course of the day and NEVER pass breakfast. This isn't a allow to stuff yourself, though – definitely honor your starvation and definitely placed down the fork while you are glad.

You will discover that on a plant-primarily based totally weight loss program, you could want to devour pretty a piece extra in quantity than you is probably used to on the way to get in enough energy for ideal adrenal function – that is due to the fact plant ingredients are full of fiber and water, while processed ingredients are regularly incorporate concentrated 'empty energy' encumbered with processed oil and delicate sugar. A healthy bean salad might also additionally incorporate lesser energy than a small, greasy pastry, for example. Every individual's consumption could be different, however try and intention for at the least the equal quantity of energy which you have been consuming previous to switching to complete ingredients, or maybe extra in case you have been proscribing.

When you first begin getting rid of addictive, processed meals from your weight loss program, you could discover you continue to having cravings for them withinside the beginning. Whilst you're scuffling with those cravings, don't be afraid to load up your plate with wholesome plant ingredients, and snack regularly. The extra glad you're, the much less probabilities you may attain for that bag of chips!

Sweets and Treats
If you discover you're yearning sweets, as a lot of us with Adrenal Fatigue do, choose complete meals with herbal sugars which include complete culmination. Instead of subtle white sugar, you could update with more healthy sweeteners in moderation (reduce for the duration of the early degrees of your recuperation process), which include coconut sugar, natural maple syrup, stevia, dates or natural date syrup. Avoid the usage of synthetic chemical sweeteners, that may wreak havoc to your fitness and metabolism.

Also watch out that a few cereals, breads, dressings and condiments can regularly incorporate white sugar, every so often in fantastically massive amounts, so make certain to test labels and pick out merchandise with healthy ingredients. Choose excessive pleasant bread made with complete grains (gluten loose is best), in preference to processed, white flour. Opt for gluten loose herbal oats, puffed brown rice or quinoa flakes, for example, crowned with sparkling culmination and seeds as a substitute than

pretty processed cereals containing sugar.

Salt Surprise
Healthy adrenal characteristic calls for sodium, and sodium is commonly low in the ones struggling Adrenal Fatigue. Unless you're an man or woman with Adrenal Fatigue and excessive blood pressure, it's now no longer an amazing concept to restriction your salt consumption. Be positive now no longer to overdo it either – a pinch or introduced to food is adequate, and pick out excessive pleasant sea salt. Celtic or Himalayan sea salt are fantastic selections due to the fact additionally they incorporate different crucial minerals and vitamins that the processing of conventional desk salt has removed.

Ditch the Dairy
Commercial dairy merchandise are pasteurized, which makes the protein withinside the dairy product extra hard to digest. This ends in extra infection withinside the frame. How does the frame reply to extended infection? The adrenal glands produce cortisol. Bingo. Avoiding dairy merchandise enables lessen infection, which enables the adrenal glands dangle directly to its cortisol.

According to Dr. Michael Greger (doctor and across the world identified fitness and nutrients speaker), the intake of dairy merchandise has additionally been connected to diverse hormonal imbalances, acne, excessive cholesterol, cancer, coronary heart disorder and diabetes, simply to call a few – yep, even diabetes. We are regularly misinformed that sugar (even from herbal sources) is the reason of insulin problems, while in reality, an extra of saturated fats determined in animal merchandise (dairy, eggs and meat) creates extra acidity withinside the frame, decreasing its cappotential to modify insulin levels. This is a horrific information for anyone, specifically the ones people with Adrenal Fatigue with already hindered insulin regulation. Why positioned your fitness at risk? Reduce your consumption of animal merchandise and make the easy transfer over to natural milk alternatives, like almond, rice or coconut, if you're looking for a milk-kind beverage.

Go Organic

Many with Adrenal Fatigue Syndrome can't tolerate the pesticides, herbicides, antibiotics or different chemical substances sprayed onto or fed into our meals as it's far grown or produced. Eating natural produce anyplace feasible enables lessen our poisonous load. Consuming natural ocean vegetables, like seaweed, enables to offer hint iodine, which helps thyroid characteristic.

Stay Hydrated

Fluid "dis-regulation" is a not unsualplace hassle in Adrenal Fatigue. The adrenalin launched while the frame is beneathneath strain will increase the fee of urine flow, and in line with Dr. Michael Lam, maximum Adrenal Fatigue patients are in a few level of fluid depletion or dehydration.

Make sure you are consuming enough spring or filtered water (a better option than tap water which may be chlorinated and fluoridated in many municipal water systems) to help your body maintain fluid balance. As a general guide, you should try to drink an ounce of water for each pound you weigh, per day (approximately 33ml per kilogram).

Additionally, eating sparkling coconut water (typically cited as "nature's Gatorade") additionally works efficaciously in hydrating and replenishing electrolytes.

Steer Clear of Stimulants

Omit stimulants which include caffeine, cacao, strength drinks, drugs, and alcohol. The short-time period improve you experience is destructive on your recovery. They activate your adrenals to make cortisol and adrenalin, mimicking the 'combat or flight' strain response, that is simply including to the weight to your worn-out adrenals. Try changing cacao (or cocoa) with powdered carob if growing your very own healthful treats. Carob makes a extraordinary stimulant-loose opportunity for the devoted chocoholic.

Green tea is appropriate in moderation, which you can drink in alternative of your ordinary cup of espresso to assist ditch the addiction and reduce caffeine cravings. It ought to be recognized that espresso is likewise a diuretic, that means it removes water from your frame inflicting dehydration. Coffee is likewise acidic, and may be aggravating to the belly and disappointed digestion, and as a stimulant can hold you wakeful at night (to the detriment on your adrenals).

Teas Between Meals

Another extremely good manner to hydrate and offer your frame with nutrition, in particular among meals, is to brew and drink caffeine free, entire leaf, natural natural teas. Not black tea, because of its caffeine content, however teas with excessive antioxidant and anti inflammatory qualities. Some splendid teas for adrenal aid consist of licorice tea, hibiscus (flor de Jamaica), that is full of antioxidants and nutrition C, and rooibos (or crimson tea), which has

been studied to ease the signs of strain and decrease strain hormone ranges. Coldwater steeping can also additionally bring about higher concentrations of vitamins than warm steeping, especially for hibiscus tea. Dandelion tea is likewise full of nutrients and minerals, and dandelion 'espresso' is a extremely good alternative for folks who are lacking the wealthy flavor in their ordinary espresso fix. Consume teas with warning in case you are pregnant.

Timing of Meals

Eating quickly after you have up is one of the maximum critical modifications you could make in addressing your Adrenal Fatigue. Overnight, your blood sugar ranges drop, and the longer you wait withinside the morning to consume a nutritious breakfast, the larger the call for you're putting to your adrenals to pressure your frame with out meals. Breakfast inside half-hour of waking is ideal. If you could't belly that, breakfast ought to be ate up in the hour.

An early lunch is likewise critical, due to the fact your frame will burn via its breakfast pretty quickly. The nice time for lunch is among 11:30am and 12pm. Also intention for a strong snack among 2 and three pm that will help you trip via the cortisol low that we realize is coming among three and 4.

Aim for a night meal among five and six pm, and plan for a excessive high-satisfactory snack approximately 30-forty five mins earlier than mattress that will help you climate sleep disturbances. (I will communicate greater approximately sleep withinside the subsequent chapter.)

Snacking

Those stricken by Adrenal Fatigue often have hassle keeping blood sugar ranges. Yes, your blood check outcomes can also additionally display normal, however you can nonetheless showcase symptoms and symptoms of hypoglycemia: dizziness, anxiety, fatigue, and every so often even a experience of being drowned. Healthy common snacking is one of the nice methods to dispose of those signs. Get into the addiction of wearing a snack with you anywhere you go. Taking a nutritious snack simply earlier than mattress may assist you nod off easier, and live asleep, due to the fact your blood sugar is in higher balance. Here are a few healthful Adrenal Fatigue snacking suggestions:

- Slightly salted snacks are helpful, as those with Adrenal Fatigue Syndrome are often in a salt depletion state because of the aldosterone dysregulation.
- Nuts – organic and raw tree nuts, like almonds, walnuts, cashews, pistachios, macadamias or pecans. Peanuts are not actually nuts, they're from the legume family, and in addition to being a common allergen they can also cause internal inflammation. Sorry peanut butter fans, no peanuts during the initial stages of your healing process.
- Organic and raw trail mix.
- Fresh fruits including apples, pears, berries, cherries, mango, stone fruit or bananas to sustain energy levels.
- Organic dried fruits, once your Adrenal Fatigue is stabilized, including goji berries, cranberries, blueberries, mulberries and goldenberries.
- Plain, unbuttered popcorn with sea salt.
- Hummus (made with organic tahini) and fresh vegetables like carrots, celery or bell peppers.
- Wholegrain crackers (could be made from brown rice, corn or quinoa) topped with avocado, tomato, radish, sea salt and pepper.

Help Heal the Adrenals with These Foods

Seaweeds (kelp, wakame, nori, kombu, dulse)
- Sprouts and leafy greens
- Whole food carbohydrates
- Whole fats in moderation, such as avocado and coconut
- Berries
- Carob
- Sea salt
- Miso, fermented naturally without MSG
- Red and orange vegetables
- Cruciferous vegetables, broccoli, cauliflower, kale
- Vegetable juices
- Ginger
- Almonds, chia seeds and flaxseeds
- Beans and legumes, when combined with wholegrain foods, and
- Licorice tea.

Avoid Foods that Hurt Adrenals

- Coffee and black tea

- Refined sugars
- Alcohol
- Deep-fried anything
- Processed foods
- Saturated fats, including meat, cheese and eggs
- Addictive fast food and junk food
- Any food to which you are sensitive or allergic
- Milk and dairy products
- Products containing highly refined flours (pasta, bread, cookies, pies, cakes, etc)
- Gluten (limit where possible or eliminate if you are sensitive)
- Chocolate (containing cacao, cocoa, dairy or sugar)
- Rancid oils, nuts and seeds (even 'good' oils go bad, often quickly), and
- Artificial sweeteners, artificial ingredients.

Supplements and Herbal Support

Common errors in Adrenal Fatigue restoration consist of the use of dietary dietary supplements and prescription medicinal drugs improperly, regularly taking an excessive amount of which could upload more pressure at the frame. Vitamin dietary supplements and natural drugs ought to most effective be utilized in live performance with the pointers on this ee-e book for a healthful, balanced diet, and in no way alternatively for healthful eating.

It is likewise critical to hold in thoughts that dietary dietary supplements aren't regulated, And there are unethical manufacturers available who're greater interested by income extent and income than your wellbeing. As well, loss of investment for research into capability poisonous effects approach there's little to no "general dosage" information. And, how one individual responds to at least one dose of a dietary or natural complement may be pretty one-of-a-kind from another.

Okay, now let's test a number of the nutrients and herbs which have assisted many human beings in recuperating from Adrenal Fatigue. You can acquire a number of the nutrients and minerals referred to from herbal meals sources, aleven though a few extra supplementation can also additionally assist make stronger your healing

process.

Herbal Remedies
Herbal medicinal drug is older than civilization. Animals of a wide variety will intentionally consume precise plant life as a manner to cope with viruses, bacteria, worms or parasites. History tells us that Aboriginal and Chinese healers going returned millennia have regarded to the plant life furnished with the aid of using Mother Nature to heal and hold the frame in balance.

Here are a number of the maximum common, and effective, herbs which might be useful in addressing Adrenal Fatigue.

Licorice Root (Glycyrrhizin Glabra and G. Uralensis)
Licorice is broadly used to deal with Adrenal Insufficiency in addition to ulcers. It enables impact the stability of cortisone and cortisol withinside the frame. Adrenal blessings may be located with simply small doses of licorice, approximately 25 – seventy five mg of standardized extract in keeping with day. Available in pill or liquid extract form, licorice use is said to have progressed fitness blessings withinside the regions of blood sugar control, higher absorption of iron, decreased inflammation, progressed hormone stability in girls, and restoration of the liner of the gut. *(Note that licorice isn't always associated with anise, big name anise, or fennel, no matter the taste similarities. When seeking out a licorice natural supplement, make sure you are becoming the actual aspect and now no longer a product made with the much less high priced anise.)*

Ginkgo Leaf (Ginkgo Biloba)

It is normally regarded that Ginkgo enables enhance flow, however it may actually have a useful effect on pressure levels. For hundreds of years, the Chinese have extensively utilized Ginkgo for some of problems from bronchial allergies and libido help to anti-aging. Ginkgo is likewise related to useful mind characteristic results like extended alertness and memory, and decreased mind fog and intellectual fatigue.

Ginkgo mainly enables with Adrenal Fatigue thru its anti-oxidative properties, which assist shield the adrenals from capacity unfastened radical damage.

Again, now no longer all Ginkgo merchandise are the identical fine. Look for standardized extracts with 24 percentage ginkgo flavones and glycosides, and six percentage bilobalides and ginkgolides. Ginkgo is likewise to be had in liquid or pill form.

Korean Ginseng Root (Panax Ginseng)

Western natural medication practitioners use the primary root of the Korean Ginseng plant to deal with bodily or intellectual exhaustion. However, in conventional Chinese medication it's miles used to sell durability and give a boost to essential electricity. Recent research have supported using Korean Ginseng root to help with insulin sensitivity, higher blood flow withinside the mind, progressed immune gadget and alleviation from a few signs and symptoms of menopause. If you've got got problems with sleep disturbances, it isn't always endorsed which you take Panax Ginseng any later than midday.

Siberian Ginseng Root (Eleutherococus Senticosus)

Sometimes referred to as Eleuthero, this herb enables with intellectual processing, immune characteristic and pressure. What's surely occurring is that the Siberian Ginseng Root acts like a slight stressor to the frame, and it's the frame's very own reaction to the pressure that money owed for the said healing blessings. For this reason, simplest people with slight Adrenal Fatigue must use this herb quick time period to keep away from overwhelming the frame's pressure reaction gadget similarly and aggravating the circumstance over time.

Ashwagandha (Withania Somnifera)

This is an historical Indian herb that has been broadly utilized by India's Ayurvedic physicians for some of healing purposes, together with progressed characteristic of the adrenal glands. Ashwagandha is a substance that enables the frame go back to everyday. If cortisol is simply too high, taking Ashwagandha will assist decrease it. If cortisol is simply too low, Ashwagandha will assist boom it. Taking Ashwagandha proper earlier than bedtime can assist enhance the fine of sleep for a few people.

Ginger Root (Zingiber Officinale)
Ginger root enables carry blood stress and coronary heart charge returned into everyday ranges, ends in extended electricity and metabolic charge, which in flip enables to burn fat. It is likewise said to stimulate digestive enzyme secretions that assist the frame take in proteins and fatty acids.

Those with diabetes, liver disorder or alcohol dependence must use warning the use of ginger root. Liquid arrangements of ginger root regularly incorporate alcohol and/or sugar. In a few arrangements, ginger root additionally incorporates aristolochic acid, which might also additionally result in kidney or urinary gadget disorder. Signs consist of blood withinside the urine or an uncommon extrade in the quantity of urine produced.

Pregnant or breast-feeding girls must additionally keep away from the use of ginger root merchandise.

A Note About Stimulating Effects
If you observe extended electricity and much less fatigue while taking any of the above natural supplements, you will be tempted to celebrate. However, as talked about with the aid of using Dr. Michael Lam, the extra reported you experience this stimulation, the extra excessive your Adrenal Fatigue, and you could surely be similarly depleting your adrenals as they paintings more difficult to preserve the inspired state. If you enjoy sizeable stimulation or another uncommon facet impact you must reduce returned and modify your amounts.

Vitamins and Minerals
There are some of nutrition and mineral dietary supplements that could assist guide adrenal feature. Not all of those indexed dietary supplements may be suitable or essential for every character, so that you may also select to devour them via mild meals reassets instead. The effects of your saliva and different exams will assist you and your fitness practitioner, when you have one, decide which of those dietary supplements can be proper for you.

Vitamin C
Vitamin C is one of the key nutrients that could significantly help recuperation from Adrenal Fatigue. It's an antioxidant that works

immediately with the adrenals to provide cortisol. Vitamin C additionally complements absorption of iron to assist fight anemia. In addition, it's widely recognized to assist improve the immune device and guard towards loose radicals. 1000mcg is a great beginning dose. Look for liposomal or buffered nutrition C.

Food reassets: Raspberries, sprouts, papaya, kiwi, inexperienced leafy vegetables, tomatoes, hibiscus tea, citrus fruits, strawberries, amla (gooseberry) powder, citrus fruit, broccoli, purple or yellow bell peppers.

B Vitamins
B12, B6 and B5 all make contributions to mobile metabolic feature. Taking excessive pleasant B dietary supplements can assist improve electricity. Specifically, B12 allows with mobile restore and purple blood mobile maintenance; B6 allows create adrenal hormones; B5 allows wreck down proteins, carbs and fat. Aim for baseline doses of a hundred mcg of B12, 50mg of B6, and 1000mg of B5.

Food reassets: Nutritional yeast, brewers yeast, nuts, miso, entire grains, potato, avocado, soybeans (and edamame), bananas, lentils.

Magnesium
Studies endorse that as many as seventy five percentage of Americans are magnesium deficient, with produces signs and symptoms of fatigue, depression, insomnia and muscle cramping. Too lots magnesium can produce digestive problems, so begin with a four hundred mg dose to ensure you may tolerate it.

Food reassets: Sesame seeds (or tahini), quinoa, pumpkin seeds, kidney beans, spinach, almonds, tempeh, inexperienced vegetables, wild rice, dates, flaxseed.

Selenium
Selenium is an essential hint mineral this is critical for wholesome thyroid and adrenal feature and additionally protects from mobile damage. Ingesting an excessive amount of selenium may be toxic, so in case you select to take a complement, attempt no greater than 2 hundred mcg each couple of days, temporarily, all through your recovery manner.

Food reassets: Mustard, brown rice, brazil nuts, cabbage, chia seeds, arrowroot powder, mushrooms, onions, sunflower seeds.

Probiotics

Probiotics assist enhance digestion, which allows the frame manner greater of the vitamins in our meals. They additionally offer immune device guide. Look for a dairy loose probiotic complement that has at the least five lines of bacteria, such as Lactobacillus acidophilus DDS-1, and 10 billion CFUs (colony forming units).

Food reassets: Sauerkraut, kimchi, kombucha tea, miso, pickles, olives, nut milks.

Other Helpful Supplements
These compounds can be useful and are all without problems to be had on line and at maximum pharmacies or fitness meals stores. Try Omega-3 (non-fish and plant- derived) to assist lessen inflammation, CoQ10 to provide electricity and hold cell feature, Acetyl-L-Carnitine to enhance metabolism, and a plant- derived Vitamin D complement in case you aren't absorbing at the least 15 mins of daylight every day.

CHAPTER 6
Curing Adrenal Fatigue Naturally: Sleep, Rest & Exercise

Sleep, relaxation and workout all play key roles in dealing with and recuperating from pressure. Even workout – generally touted as a obligatory detail in accurate fitness – can purpose greater pressure if now no longer executed correctly on your character degree of adrenal fitness. Falling via the cracks among sleep and workout is relaxation. Simple relaxation. I agree with that every one 3 want to accept same precedence for your adrenal fatigue recuperation plan.

Sleep and Sleep Hygiene
How is your sleep? The significance of doing all you may to make sure you get adequate, restful and restorative sleep can't be overstated. Too a lot of us have allow sleep take the backseat to different existence priorities. We have evolved bedtime behavior that get withinside the manner of right and restful sleep. Whether the end result is Adrenal Fatigue, or simply perpetual exhaustion, listening to sleep hygiene could make a large difference.

What is Sleep Hygiene?

Sleep hygiene is a time period used to explain some of practices that assist make sure that midnight is complete of pleasant sleep, and daylight hours is complete of alertness. The maximum essential of all of the practices is to set up a regular, 7-day-per- week, sleep and wake pattern. Not a Monday-Friday pattern, and some other for the weekends. This includes spending the proper quantity of time in bed. Here is a listing of encouraged and wholesome sleep hygiene practices:

- Discipline yourself to reserve your bed for the two "s" activities, sex and sleep. Avoid watching TV, working on your laptop, or even reading.
- Eliminate caffeine, nicotine and alcohol. Alcohol may help you get to sleep, but as your body starts to metabolize the alcohol it wakes you up and disrupts your sleep.
- Exercise: vigorous exercise is okay in the morning or afternoon, *IF* this doesn't cause an adrenal crash, but restrict evening exercise to relaxing forms of activity like yoga (I'll get into exercise in more detail shortly).
- Make sure you get enough natural light. If you have been cooped up inside, whether due to winter or illness, find a way to expose yourself to some sunshine – the 'happy' vitamin. This additionally facilitates the frame apprehend the distinction among day and night time and beef up the message that daylight is for waking and midnight for sleep.
- No daytime napping. It can disrupt the important circadian rhythm of the sleep-wakeful cycles.
- Don't eat too close to bedtime, and remember that any changes in your diet may trigger sleep problems.
- Set up a bedtime routine that is relaxing. Avoid emotionally upsetting conversations just before you are going to sleep.
- Restrict the use of electronics in the half hour before bed and eliminate them in bed. The light from the bright screens works to trick your brain into thinking it is daytime. At the very least, put your screen on the dimmest possible setting if you must use the device in the evening hours leading to bedtime.

Rest, Relax and Reduce Stress

Rest, relaxation after which relaxation a few greater. Once you've achieved that, discover a precise spot to take a seat down or lie down, and relaxation. Okay, I jest. But only a little.

Examine the manner you've got got been undertaking your life, and word how normally in the course of an afternoon you "push on through" due to the fact you suspect you've got got to "get matters achieved". This is conduct that has contributed in your condition, and also you should stop. Taking a 5-minute spoil among duties isn't always going to make a vast dent on your productivity, however it's miles going that will help you reclaim your fitness.

Managing Stress

Stress is regularly considered as some thing that takes place "to" us, some thing this is past our control. With that perspective, we're victims, powerless to

extrade how strain influences us. If this resonates with you, and sounds authentic for you, I actually have news.

You do have the electricity to select your reaction to the outside event. Mindfulness sporting events may be very useful in coaching a way to separate the "judgments" we observe to almost each situation, thought, action, and manner in our lives from the matters themselves. This facilitates to lessen the emotional responses, regularly stressful, and lets in us to view matters greater objectively.

Worrying is an example. Decide to have a high-quality mind-set and regularly a listing of concerns shrinks considerably. Ask your self if the problem is some thing inside your control, or outdoor your control? If it's some thing this is past your control, pass it off the listing. Worrying is harming your fitness. If it absolutely is a choice you should make, attempt creating a word of it or write approximately it in a journal, and placed it away for some other time. But now no longer simply earlier than bed, wherein it'll intrude together along with your sleep.

Look for methods to shift your views and attitudes on life, as necessary. Examples encompass training gratitude, appreciation, letting go, forgiveness, and exploring spirituality. All of those are effective adjustments that produce high-quality extrade in how your frame and mind experience – and perceive – strain.

Breathing – the Building Block of Successful Stress Management

Most of the time we're subconscious approximately our breath. It takes place automatically. One of the simplest matters you could do as you begin at the route to healing from Adrenal Fatigue Syndrome is to exercise deep, slow, clean and rhythmic breathing, the use of the diaphragm.

This facilitates launch anxiety from the frame, facilitates clean the mind, reduces fatigue and improves each intellectual and bodily wellness.

Balance Your Life
Too a whole lot paintings, an excessive amount of doing matters for others, and too little time to attend to your self. That's a recipe that has to extrade so as to your healing to have a shot at success.

Get Rid of Energy Suckers
We've all acknowledged folks that appear to suck electricity out of the room whenever

they're around. Got a person like that during your life? These human beings are electricity- robbers, and also you don't have sufficient electricity to go 'round. Avoid them, even though most effective temporarily.

Happiness and Connections
And did you recognize that happiness is a skill, in place of an attribute? Psychology professor and happiness researcher Sonja Lyubomirsky explains that most effective approximately 50 percentage of a person's happiness is genetic. And of that 50, most effective 10 percentage is due to fitness, earnings and looks. Still, there's an entire 50 percentage that may be a found out skill.

Research tells us that one of the most powerful signs of happiness and precise fitness is the nice and electricity of our human connections. Relationships and family, yes, however I'm speaking approximately network connections too. If you examine this and recognize which you've been spending all of your time being concerned to your youngsters and cleansing the house, or giving the entirety you've were given to the workplace 12 hours an afternoon, and also you infrequently spend any time certainly connecting with human beings on your network, now could be the time to begin. What approximately your paintings connections? They may be beneficial, however if the ones are the most effective connections you've were given on your life, it's really well worth taking some other look. Take a class. Join a club. Check out a community truthful or event. Find some thing that pursuits you, even a little, that your contemporary agenda doesn't appear to permit.

Go in advance and create time for a few romance, for a few a laugh with buddies and family, and go away the guilt experience locked withinside the basement.

Look for methods to spend quiet time together along with your self. Treat your self to a bath, a walk, or a manicure, some thing which you experience, after which permit your self to experience it!

Lighten Up With Laughter

Laughter is one of the excellent sports for converting the manner we sense.

Studies display that folks that snicker frequently have decrease tiers of cortisol and epinephrine, decrease blood pressure, and decrease emotions of tension and strain. The research additionally recommend that even faking laughter is beneficial: the frame doesn't seem like capin a position to differentiate among the actual aspect and a synthetic snicker. No joking!

So, cross ahead. Let your self snicker, even though it's miles at your self.

Exercise

It may be so confusing. On one hand, we realize that we should get our coronary heart quotes up – aerobic – to be able to stave off coronary heart disease. On the alternative hand, we realize that exercising can precipitate an adrenal crash. We've been bombarded with messages approximately the significance of "operating up a sweat", and we had been conditioned to assume that if we haven't genuinely "driven ourselves to the limit", it wasn't genuinely treasured exercising.

With Adrenal Fatigue Syndrome, you want to regulate all of that thinking. Exercise without a doubt has an vital function in recovery, however you need to create a method this is suitable to the extent of Adrenal Fatigue Syndrome you're struggling with. Doing the incorrect type of exercising, at the incorrect depth stage, can cause every other crash instead of assist you get better.

The trick is to layout a method and method that builds a customised application this is appropriate in your unique stage of Adrenal Fatigue Syndrome.

Stop Intense Exercise

That's proper. Stop any in depth shape of exercising for at the least a month, longer if needed. Take a smash from aerobic and all different types of strenuous exercising.

Restorative Exercise

Many humans with Adrenal Fatigue Syndrome will enjoy crashes brought on via way of means of everyday stretching and strengthening exercising, that is regularly considered "mild" withinside the bodily health world.

Adrenal restorative exercising is extraordinary, designed to assist locate stability and repair fitness via way of means of connecting the thoughts and frame in a nurturing and restorative manner. If your Adrenal Fatigue is withinside the early ranges, stage one or, you can have achievement in restorative yoga classes. For people with extra superior Adrenal Fatigue, even restorative yoga can be an excessive amount of and cause a crash.

Regular, Light Exercise
As you begin to heal, you may probable locate you sense excellent with strolling or mild cycling. Do now no longer overstress your frame with strenuous sports.

You can also additionally locate your self absolutely tired after exercising, and as a end result you've

found out to keep away from it altogether. Completely understandable, however besides throughout an adrenal crash, it's now no longer a great concept to absolutely forgo any shape of exercising.

CHAPTER 7
The Road to Recovery

Adrenal Fatigue can soak up to 10 years or extra to manifest, so it's miles vital which you assume it to make an effort to resolve, after you get at the proper street to recovery.

Don't be discouraged in case you don't shed pounds immediately. You should keep in mind that an Adrenal Fatigued frame has continued a extremely good deal of strain and should heal first. Your organs and hormones want to be operating optimally so as for weight reduction to occur. A gradual launch of weight will permit time in your frame to rebuild and agree with itself once more and, as a end result, you may maintain the load off withinside the lengthy run. Be affected person and sort to your self, and permit weight reduction to take place naturally.

You can also additionally sense tempted to have a good time and loosen up after you begin feeling better, however maintain going! Your new life-style conduct are operating. As time is going on, you could progressively lessen your dosage of dietary dietary supplements and preserve your newfound fitness via the strength of life-style and diet.

Recovery Process

Recovery pace and system is extraordinary for almost anyone with AFS. Depending at the severity of your unique condition, different fitness implications, and your willingness to change, your system may take some weeks, some months, or maybe longer.

Preparation Phase

This coaching length is crucial for lengthy-time period achievement.

- 1 day to 6 weeks depending on the level of AFS
- May be no noticeable improvement in symptoms even though nutrients are changing for the better
- Reactions to nutrients may arise, resulting in feeling worse, adjustments need to be made
- Body is in process of healing and resetting internally.

Honeymoon Phase

- A few days to 12 weeks or more depending on level of AFS
- Body handles stress better, reduced fatigue, anxiety noticeably diminishes, sleep improves
- Can be mini-crashes and setbacks, don't despair, recovery from these should be quicker than before you embarked on your recovery road
- Energy begins to return.

Plateau Phase

It's sincerely not possible to set a time body for this length. It may be some weeks or some months. It should final for years and you may be absolutely symptom free, in case you have been in stage one or of AFS.

But the truth stays that the frame should have time to rebuild itself, and for the ones in stage 3 or four, the extra superior ranges of AFS, this truly takes as lots time because it takes.

It is viable that the ones of you with extra extreme AFS can also additionally want to slowly adapt to a decrease stage of normal strength function.

Expect Ongoing Cycles

Recovery isn't linear. Like healing from addiction, foremost surgery, or some other foremost illness, the direction of healing is cyclical. Expect a spiral, and face up to the frustration or depression while you all at once sense like you've suffered a setback.

I'll say it again: cyclical mini crashes and recoveries are to be expected.

The maximum dramatic and substantial development might be in early tiers of treatment. Then, after a length of time, you'll all at once understand that the setbacks have become much less severe, that they don't closing as long, and over time, that the durations among those mini-crashes receives longer. You'll word that your highs might be highly higher, your lows now no longer as low.

Cycles, like a spiral, a touch development, a touch setback. Normal.

Willingness to Change

All the pleasant clinical recommendation and assist withinside the international will do really no right in case you don't observe the pointers. If you maintain together along with your negative weight loss plan habits, don't observe thru at the workout pointers (both to workout greater, or much less, relying to your degree of AFS), and fail to take the advised supplements, you'll now no longer see any development to your Adrenal Fatigue.

It additionally takes a willingness to pinpoint and remove the reassets of pressure to your life. This may be extraordinarily difficult, on occasion requiring the termination of long-status relationships, leaving a job, or converting your dating with money.

Not all people reveals they're able to making the desire - deciding on their fitness and well being over the fame quo - however in case you do, you'll attain the rewards, sense better, have greater power and pleasure to your life. Speaking from private experience, it's miles really well worth it.

Remember, you DESERVE to get well, and also you DESERVE the time and power to make it happen.

Feeling Like Yourself Again

If making a decision to stroll down the street to healing, and you're taking to coronary heart the tips, tips and pointers on this book, I recognize you'll begin to sense better.

You can have your libido back, your power back, you can lose a few extra weight, and you'll once more have the power and motivation to get thru your day.

I actually have travelled this street myself, and feature for my part attempted the whole lot I recommend right here and greater. I actually have researched and attempted lots greater than is captured on this book, and I actually have discovered what appears to work, what doesn't, and what's sincerely a waste of time.

I thanks for taking the time to examine this book, and I want you each achievement and right fitness.

CHAPTER 8
Bonus Adrenal Support Recipes

Please experience those plant-based, complete meals recipes. They are amongst my favorites, and are actually staples in my weight loss plan. These recipes, and others, have helped me get over Adrenal Fatigue and are at the least partially liable for my ongoing right fitness.

Smoothies and Tea

Banana, Berry and Chia Smoothie
Ingredients

Directions

  ½ cup frozen wild blueberries
  ½ cup frozen strawberries
  ½ frozen banana
  1 cup baby spinach 1 cup
  almond milk 1tsp. chia seeds

knife comes away clean.
11.   Makes 12 muffins.

Vegan Strawberry Banana 'Nice' Cream
(No ice cream maker required)

Ingredients

Directions

1 cup frozen strawberries
3 ripe frozen bananas (very ripe and frozen at least 24 hours) 2 T coconut
milk (other nut milks work too but coconut is my fave for this)
2T shredded coconut
4 small fresh mint leaves

1. Using the "S" or dough blade of your meals processor, combination strawberries with the coconut milk till you've were given texture like sorbet.
2. Add bananas and preserve mixing till properly mixed, fluffy and creamy.
3. Serve immediately, or keep withinside the freezer.
   4. Sprinkle shredded coconut and upload a mint sprig on pinnacle of every character serving.
   5. Makes four servings.

Easy Date and Nut Energy Bars

Ingredients

Directions

- 2 cups medjool dates, pitted and chopped into satisfactory chunks
- ½ cup mixed chopped nuts (walnuts, pecans, almonds, macadamia)
- 3 T coconut flakes
- A palm full of chopped, dried fruit of choice (optional)

1. Heat non-stick skillet over medium heat. Add coconut flakes, tossing or stirring constantly till golden brown. Watch carefully – the flakes pass from brown to burnt in seconds.
2. Mash chopped dates in blending bowl, then stir in nuts, dried fruit and coconut. If you decide on crumb-sized pieces, you could pulse all substances in a meals processor.
3. Pour blend into baking dish, covered with plastic wrap, urgent to approximately ¾ inch thick.
4. Refrigerate at the least 1/2 of an hour.
5. To cast off from the dish, pull up at the plastic wrap.
6. Remove the wrap, and reduce bars to preferred size.
7. Can be re-wrapped and saved withinside the fridge and used as grab'n'pass snack, brief breakfast, or dessert.

CHAPTER 1
Herbs

Ginkgo Biloba

Gingko Biloba is an historic and fast-developing Chinese tree with a protracted records of medicinal use withinside the East. In fact, it would also be the oldest surviving tree species at the earth; professionals have dated it again a mind- boggling three hundred million years. Can you accept as true with it?

It works to enhance your mind and intellectual overall performance on many degrees. Firstly, it improves the blood waft on your mind, flooding the tissues with oxygen and enhancing reminiscence and attention withinside the process.

It's additionally supremely excessive in antioxidants, which could shield the mind from the harm of loose radicals, age-associated reminiscence decline and additionally Alzheimer's disease.

Gingko additionally has a big impact upon melancholy and coffee temper disorders. The flavonoids it includes are referred to as terpene lactones and ginkgo-flavone glycosides (flavonoids) which assist preserve degrees of dopamine and serotonin to your mind, and in flip enhance each temper and idea processes.

It comes in lots of exclusive forms - tablets, tincture or even tea form. Take among eighty mg and 240 mg in step with day, divided into at the least doses. It's exceptional to take the primary dose after breakfast and the second one after lunch, to make sure that you may nonetheless drop off to sleep at night. Be conscious that it is able to absorb to twelve weeks for the outcomes of gingko to end up apparent. Be patient.

Ginseng

Ginseng has been utilized by tens of thousands and thousands of human beings over time to reinforce their
attention, enhance their reminiscence and beat dementia and Alzheimer's disease.

Not most effective this, however ginseng is a exquisite adaptogen; a treatment that objectives the outcomes of physical, emotional and environmental pressure which could result in unwell fitness and disease. It works through decreasing degrees of cortisol withinside the blood movement and strengthening adrenal glands which could frequently end up fatigued throughout hard instances in our lives.

Ginseng additionally incorporates excessive ranges of antioxidants, which assist shield our brains from the ravages of free-radicals, enhance your capacity to pay attention and can even goal signs of ADHD and short-time period reminiscence loss in all ages.

You can experience ginseng as a pill, tablet or at the same time as a tea. Take 240 mg every day to look high-quality effects.

Kava Kava

Kava Kava is the critical factor withinside the well-known South Pacific Tea Ceremony, and works wonders on strain, tension, despair, migraine or even leprosy, in line with a few sources.

In South Pacific groups it's used a lot withinside the equal manner as alcohol is used in lots of countries. Its energy lies withinside the presence of kava-lactones, that are a outstanding muscle relaxant, and come up with that chilled-out, non violent feeling that simply isn't matched with the aid of using some other anti-tension substance. It's a splendidly soothing treatment, which facilitates dissolve tension, insomnia and strain.

However, there has these days been a few problem that it may motive liver harm in positive individuals, a declare that has now no longer been substantiated with the aid of using any of the research performed to research those meant side-effects.
Communities all over the global hold to apply kava kava to sense happier, at peace and carry out at their high-quality, and you could too.

The conventional shape to devour kava kava is of route as a tea, however you could additionally get it in pill or tablet shape. Take 210-240 mg every day. Be conscious that it does have an effect on different medicines you is probably taking and it isn't always to be taken with the aid of using pregnant or breastfeeding women, or people with liver harm.

St. John's Wort

St John's Wort is a herb that grows wild withinside the meadows and roadsides of Europe and North America. It's a effective conventional treatment that has visible a latest surge in achievement because of its capacity to assist deal with despair and additionally the sunshine-poor ailment SAD (Seasonal Affective Disorder). If you want an natural pick-me-up, you couldn't pass some distance incorrect with St John's Wort.

Its energetic factor is hypericin, a polyphenol, which facilitates improve ranges of serotonin withinside the mind, main to decreased tension and higher sleep.

Studies have proven that it really works correctly to fight reminiscence problems, cognitive processing troubles and advanced getting to know while blended with Gingko Biloba. In tandem, they paintings to get rid of the pollution to your mind and improve the ones serotonin ranges that will help you sense positive, shrewd and in ownership of a sturdy reminiscence, and paintings greater correctly than while used separately.

The advocated dose is 30 mg Ginkgo Biloba (24% extract) and one hundred fifty mg of St John's Wort (0.3% hypericin). If you'd choose to use St John's Wort alone, intention for 300mg according to day.

Saint John's Wort interferes with a few prescription drugs for this reason it's far vital to test together along with your doctor earlier than taking this herb. Do now no longer use this herb in case you are taking any pharmaceutical anti-depressants.

Gotu Kola

Gotu Kola is a plant this is local to India and Asia and is utilized in Ayurvedic medicinal drug to deal with problems of the anxious machine and mind. Its energetic components brahmoside and brahminoside act as a slight sedative, lowering your ranges of strain and tension. It additionally facilitates to calm the critical anxious machine, permitting you to sense as though a weight has been lifted out of your shoulders.

Acting like a super-food, it boosts your mind, improves your alertness, mind feature and additionally your reminiscence. Plus it's filled with mind-wholesome nutrients
and minerals inclusive of nutrients A, G, and K and is likewise excessive in magnesium.

Enjoy it as a tea for high-quality results (it tastes much like chamomile tea). But you could additionally take it in tablet or pill shape. The advocated dose for strain alleviation and an development in overall performance 50 to 250 mg, 2 to three instances every day.

Ashwaghandha

Ashwagandha is a plant local to the Middle East and Africa and is a cousin of the tomato and the eggplant. Studies have proven that it'd additionally assist save you the onset of Alzheimer's ailment and related reminiscence loss. This is as it inhibits the formation of plaque with the mind, that can kill mind cells and result in the ailment.

Additionally, it acts as a nootropic and boosts your normal reminiscence, cognitive competencies and relieves strain all on the equal time. It works with the aid of using restricting the quantity of the strain hormone cortisol withinside the bloodstream, and additionally has an normal enjoyable and de-stimulating impact at the complete body, that can assist with situations like ADHD and Parkinson's ailment.

Its strong antioxidant movement facilitates to guard the frame towards the loose radicals which could result in neural harm and it can clearly assist to make contributions closer to their repair.

To enjoy the advantageous outcomes of ashwaghandha, you could complement with an quantity that fits you. You can begin with a dose of round three hundred- 500mg and growth to round 6,000mg according to day for more potent outcomes. Always divide your dose into as a minimum or 3 small doses at some stage in the day to useful resource absorption.

Lemon Balm

Lemon balm is a adorable lemon-scented herb with a protracted records of use in peoples medication as a nap useful resource and mild treatment for tension. Recent research have additionally determined that it possesses an fantastic cappotential to reinforce your reminiscence and enhance your performance, in particular in relation to getting to know new

data. The quality information is that many humans have it developing of their garden, so can experience its advantages proper away.

It consists of a large number of energetic elements that assist to obtain its advantages upon your grey matter. Compounds called eugenol and terpense assist to calm your muscle tissues and soothe your mind, and some other referred to as rosmarinic acid facilitates to manipulate your stages of strain earlier than it sincerely starts offevolved to take its toll.

Studies done at Northumbria University determined that a excessive percent of college students clearly executed higher grades after they supplemented with exceptional lemon balm. This become because of the movement of numerous compounds, which enhance the impact of the neurotransmitter acetylcholine. This neurotransmitter is critical to reminiscence formation and maintenance, logical concept and average cognition. So in case you need to loosen up and enhance your intelligence, lemon balm can be the proper solution.

It's quality taken as a tea, so when you have a bush developing to your garden, harvest the leaves and brew up your very own refreshing, aromatic cup. Otherwise, it can additionally be taken as a complement. Experts propose a dose of six hundred to 1,600mg lemon balm extract according to day.

Bacopa

Bacopa is an Ayurvedic herb with a protracted records of use for none apart from cognitive enhancement. In fact, latest research in Australia have showed that bacopa does certainly enhance data processing, verbal getting to know fee and average operating reminiscence.

It normally works its magic via way of means of boosting stages of the neurotransmitter serotonin, which in flip will enhance your temper and assist address tension and melancholy too. But it doesn't simply make you sense good; it additionally facilitates to save you the onset of Alzheimer's sickness and dementia too.

This takes place for the subsequent reasons:

Firstly, bacopa consists of a excessive stage of antioxidants, which offer a defensive impact upon the mind, save you loose-radical harm to the cells and anxious device and enhance average health. Secondly, bacopa facilitates to interrupt down the beta amyloid proteins which could result in plaque accumulation withinside the

mind and result in Alzheimer's sickness. And thirdly, it facilitates to heal broken mind cells and nerve cells, making it uniquely useful for the ones affected by dementia and mind harm.

To experience the advantages take round three hundred mg according to day.

Huperzia Serrata

Huperzia is a kind of moss this is local to India and South East Asia and it can be our quality wish but withinside the war towards Alzheimer's sickness and age- associated reminiscence loss. So a good deal in order that it has lately visible a surge in popularity, each in its use and research.

It works via way of means of growing stages of the vital neurotransmitter acetylcholine. This neurotransmitter regularly comes below assault via way of means of sure physical enzymes, which has the impact of lowering its stages withinside the frame and As a result stopping your mind cells from efficiently speaking with every other. As a result, your reminiscence declines, as does your cognitive performance.

Not most effective that, however it additionally facilitates to lessen the formation of plaque withinside the mind that ends in Alzheimer's sickness and dementia, and forestalls mind and nerve harm from clearly happening at all. You can in all likelihood see why the sector is so enthusiastic about this stuff!

If you're interested by locating out for your self how it may raise your mind, take a complement containing 50 to one hundred micrograms of its energetic factor huperzia A.

Rhodiola

Rhodiola is every other one of the herbs that falls into the 'adaptogen' category. It works through focused on lifestyles's stresses, together with physical, emotional and environmental stresses and boosting the immune device and different physical tactics to cope. As a end result, it has high-quality recuperation powers that we nonetheless don't understand the authentic quantity of.

It carries phenylpropanoids, that can raise intellectual overall performance and additionally calm the body, in addition to an antioxidant impact that allows to guard the mind from plaque formation that could additionally purpose Alzheimer's ailment and different kinds of dementia. And in addition to all of this, research have proven that intake of rhodiola can gradual the breakdown of the neurotransmitter acetylcholine, and as a end result should delay the onset of Alzheimer's ailment. It simply is an first-rate all-rounder this is best for pressure, grief, reminiscence issues and dementia.

It additionally has an anti-tension action, which allows to lessen tiers of cortisol, the pressure hormone, withinside the bloodstream, and helps the complete fearful device to assist make clear notion tactics, enhance intellectual calculation and normal overall performance.

Additionally, it will increase tiers of the neurotransmitter serotonin withinside the bloodstream, which maintains to enhance that glad feeling - although lifestyles isn't pretty going the manner you desired it to.

For quality results, take among one hundred and 1000mg every day, divided into doses.

Oregano

If I needed to select simply one culinary herb to take with me to a wasteland island, it might maximum virtually be oregano. It has such a lot of fitness benefits, and additionally tastes scrumptious introduced to all styles of vegetable dishes - there simply isn't something that comes close.

Oregano truly allows to adjust our mind waves, assisting us to experience greater relaxed, much less annoying and additionally study new records an awful lot quicker and greater effectively. This comes right all the way down to its lively components, *carvacrol and thymoquinone*, which boom each alpha-1 and beta-1 brainwaves.

Studies have additionally proven that it improves neurotransmitter feature, growing tiers of dopamine, serotonin and noradrenaline withinside the body - all hormones that hold melancholy and occasional temper at bay, and feeling happier and greater centered at the venture to hand as a end result.

It's a scrumptious inexperienced leafy herb that may be introduced to any dish you adore the

maximum. You also can use oregano as an critical oil. Simply pop some drops to your diffuser and revel in the uplifting heady fragrance. And lastly, you could take it as a complement too - begin with 400mg two times a day.

Rosemary

Rosemary is such an uplifting herb, and I am constantly reminded of walks throughout the hills of the Mediterranean whilst its heady fragrance hits my nostrils. It's an herb with a extremely good capacity to enhance your cognition, make you experience extremely good and additionally raise your temper and reminiscence. Better than that, it additionally definitely influences the rate and accuracy wherein you're capable of reply to a stimulus, making its have an effect on comparable to, and additionally advanced to, that of caffeine. This is due to a compound referred to as *1,8-cineole*, that can assist raise potential reminiscence. This is the sort of reminiscence you operate while you want to recollect a series of destiny tasks, together with attending a assembly or sending that crucial email.

Let's now no longer neglect about that rosemary is likewise a robust antioxidant and additionally possesses anti inflammatory properties, which combat loose radical harm withinside the mind and complements reminiscence and concentration. This is due to the presence of crucial compounds: *caffeic acid and rosemarinic acid*. It additionally carries carnosic acid - a phytochemical which allows to guard your mind from strokes and age-associated regeneration.

The quality manner to revel in rosemary is of direction to your meals and it tastes exquisite mixed with maximum vegetables, particularly the ones taken into consideration to be a part of the Mediterranean diet, together with peppers, eggplant, tomatoes and zucchini.

You also can revel in rosemary as a dried herb, an extract or whilst a tea. If you're choosing the extract, take 400mg rosemary drugs up to 3 instances a day. Pregnant and breastfeeding ladies must keep away from rosemary.

Thyme

Thyme is packed complete of these mind-pleasant omega-3's and could assist guard
your mind towards age-associated degeneration, in addition to enhancing your normal mind feature significantly. It's a penetrating and aromatic herb this is additionally excessive in diet C, iron, manganese, and iron.

It's additionally excessive in flavonoids, which include apigenin, *naringenin, luteolin,* and thymonin, making it a awesome antioxidant. And lastly, certainly considered one among its lively ingredients, *thymol,* assist us experience happier and keep ranges of vital fatty acids withinside the mind.

Thyme works brilliantly in vegetable and bean dishes, so throw it into your food to up the taste and acquire the mind-boosting blessings.

Sage

For loads of years, the reminiscence-boosting powers of sage had been thoroughly acknowledged. But it seems that that is no antique wives' tale - sage definitely is as top in your mind as they say. It allows raise the chemical messengers withinside the mind and with the aid of using doing so, improves reminiscence and basic performance.

Recent studies into the impact that sage has upon Alzheimer's ailment has proven that it additionally has a secret-weapon - it could inhibit a harmful enzyme referred to as acetylcholinesterase (AChE), which damages the mind and ends in the onset of the ailment. This additionally boosts ranges of the neurotransmitter acetylcholine and improves basic reminiscence and gaining knowledge of.

It's every other of the inexperienced leafy herbs that flavor tremendous and gives terrific anti-oxidant outcomes. One precise anti-growing old antioxidant named carnosic acid is capable of boost ranges of glutathione withinside the mind with the aid of using enhancing blood go with the drift to the cerebral arteries. Clearly top mind blood-go with the drift is vital in case you need to own splendid wondering energy.

Sage is scrumptious while delivered to soups, stews, salads, and might also be used to make dressings. Why now no longer develop a number of your very own sage in your windowsill at domestic and upload it for your meals regularly?

CHAPTER 2

Spices & Essential Oils

Ginger

Ginger is one of these spices that definitely merits extra credit score than it ever gets. Not simplest it's far warming and scrumptious, it additionally has the energy to enhance your idea procedures.

In a observe performed with the aid of using the Thailand Institute of Scientific and Technological Research, it become found that ginger appreciably progressed attention, cognitive processing and gaining knowledge of skills and not using a facet outcomes while utilized by middle-elderly women. If ginger can assist enhance the brains of those women, consider what it may do to you too.

Ginger also can assist to save you monosodium glutamate toxicity, some thing that has massive implications for the fitness of our brains. MSG as it's far usually acknowledged is a taste-enhancer, that's delivered to many varieties of processed ingredients. Worst of all, it has a poisonous impact upon our brains, and can make a contribution to the onset of age-associated reminiscence decline and dementia. What extra evidence can we want to keep away from processed ingredients as a long way as viable and keep on with wholefoods?

If you need to revel in a number of the blessings of ginger, you've got got masses of alternatives to pick from. You can upload it for your recipes, drink it as a tea or maybe take it in tablet form. It's advocated which you take among four hundred and 800mg in step with day for first-class results.

Turmeric

I'm quite positive which you've heard the hype approximately turmeric with the aid of using now - it's the
spice hailed as a miracle therapy for infinite fitness court cases and the maximum thrilling herbal preventative degree towards Alzheimer's ailment that you may begin to revel in proper now. India has an curiously low charge of Alzheimer's ailment, advised to be a end result of the excessive ranges of turmeric they consume.

The key's idea to lie in its excessive curcumin content. Curcumin is a effective antioxidant that allows to lessen plaque formation withinside the mind and battles towards loose radicals withinside the body. It's additionally a effective anti- inflammatory, which allows to heal the complete body.

And in addition to all of this, turmeric may also assist you to enhance your mind- energy, growth mind-mobileular restore procedures and enhance your reminiscence. This is due to every other compound that it contains, called aromatic-turmerone, which become proven to growth mind pastime in a observe performed in Germany.

All of this proof is proving to be definitely hopeful withinside the combat towards mind deterioration, and mind injury. Turmeric is the spice that offers curry its one of a kind vivid yellow color, so the first-class aspect you may do to acquire the blessings is to devour extra of them. If you're now no longer partial to curries - don't panic. A splendid tip is to sprinkle a small quantity of it into your meals. You'll slightly be capable of note the difference, and it won't upload even the slightest trace of spice for your meal.

Of course, you may additionally take turmeric in complement form - research have proven that a dose of 400mg of a natural curcumin works wonders on your mind, and additionally makes you experience amazing!

Black Pepper

Who could have idea that one of the maximum not unsualplace condiments additionally has a mystical impact upon our brains? It has the capacity to address low moods and make you experience without a doubt fabulous.

This is as it carries an energetic substance known as piperine, which protects the stages of the hormones serotonin and additionally dopamine withinside the mind. This has first-rate implications for despair and temper problems in addition to Parkinson's ailment, as each are related to decrease stages of the respective hormones.

Piperine additionally works to enhance attention and additionally reasoning skills.

It will increase stages of beta-endorphins withinside the mind and improves common cognitive overall performance ensuing in a happier you and a more potent mind.

You can both take a piperine complement of round 15-20mg or be beneficiant with the amount of black pepper which you upload for your foods. The preference is yours!

Cinnamon

Cinnamon's recognition as a health-boosting drug has come on in leaps and boundaries of the beyond few years, and for a first-rate cause too. Not most effective does it assist with weight loss and meals cravings, it really works miracles in your mind feature too.

It's a first-rate supply of the mineral manganese which acts as a effective anti- oxidant, defensive the frame from the ravages of loose radicals that may result in Alzheimer's, dementia and additionally cancers. It's worried in the ideal functioning of the mind, and so from a dietary standpoint, it's without a doubt perfect.

Cinnamon additionally carries compounds that assist to beat back the onset of Alzheimer's ailment. These are cinnamaldehyde and epicatechin, that may save you plaque formation withinside the mind that may result in the ailment.

Like so the various different spices, you may actually sprinkle a small amount of the spice onto your preferred food and in smoothies. You also can select a complement of round 1000mg in line with day to revel in the equal type of benefits.

Nutmeg

Eating nutmeg will maintain you as sharp as a pin! It carries a herbal natural compound known as miristicin, with a purpose to enhance your reminiscence and allows beat back loose-radical harm that would result in Alzheimer's ailment or different sorts of dementia.

If you're struggling strain and insomnia, nutmeg would possibly simply be your cure. Sprinkled right into a heat drink past due at night, it's going to assist loosen up your frame and permit you get the type of rejuvenating sleep which you deserve, in addition to lessen stages of hysteria and strain you is probably experiencing.

Nutmeg is likewise effective in important minerals which include potassium, calcium, iron and manganese which all sell healthful mind feature.

Simply upload a small quantity for your soups, stews, smoothies or maybe your oatmeal to revel in a scrumptious mind improve.

Clove

Although you won't understand it, cloves are the dried flower bud of the evergreen tree, *Eugenia aromatica*, that's local to Indonesia. They're first-class regarded for his or her pain-killing residences on the subject of toothache, however they also can assist paintings wonders on your mind too.

They're a top notch supply of omega-three oils that assist maintain your mind in tip-pinnacle condition, they're packed complete of nutrition and minerals and that they have the best meals attention of manganese out there. As a result, cloves are a first-rate supply of antioxidants, which assist solve the harm due to loose radicals and improve our whole bodies.

A observe achieved via way of means of the University College of Medical Sciences in Delhi, India found that clove oil can honestly opposite short-time period and long-time period reminiscence deficits suffered during our lives.

When used as an aromatherapy oil, clove oil additionally successfully goals strain, despair and tension via way of means of stimulating mind feature and coping with the stages of neurotransmitters and hormones withinside the blood.

You can upload floor cloves to many foods, in addition to playing it as an aromatherapy oil or remedy oil.

Sweet Orange Essential Oil

Sweet Orange Oil is one of the first-class important oils for assisting you to experience positive, uplifted and additionally creative. It's certainly considered one among my preferred important oils because it smells similar to a juicy, freshly peeled orange with the intention to go away you feeling bright, active and productive.

Its strength comes from its energetic ingredient, limonene, which has been established to lessen strain stages and assist address despair.

To use candy orange oil, genuinely integrate some drops of the natural critical oil with a tablespoon of provider oil, along with candy almond oil, and rub down into your skin. You also can use it in a diffuser to unfold the heady fragrance at some stage in the room, and permit your colleagues, pals or own circle of relatives to additionally experience its boosting benefits.

Basil Essential Oil

Basil oil has a sparkling and invigorating heady fragrance which could enhance your reminiscence, cognizance, and assist you to keep away from distraction - ideal for the ones instances if you have an critical closing date looming, or have an examination which you want to revise for.

Its lively ingredient, linalool, reduces stages of pressure and will increase stages of wellbeing, making it ideal for studying.

It has a wealthy and effective smell, so use it sparingly, both in a diffuser or through making use of a small quantity of the diluted oil for your stress factors.

Peppermint Essential Oil

Peppermint critical oil has a cooling and fresh fragrance, and for this reason it's miles broadly utilized in meals and additionally cosmetics. But did you recognize that it may additionally assist enhance the productiveness of your thoughts?

It's a outstanding opportunity to caffeine that could efficaciously address pressure, offer a outstanding feeling of whole-frame relaxation, cognizance your senses, enhance your reminiscence and awaken your thoughts, leaving you raring to go!

For first-rate effects, combo some drops of the natural critical oil with a provider oil, along with almond oil, and follow for your stress factors at some stage in the day. Of route you may additionally use it as a rub down oil, however do take care to combo it successfully as it's miles a totally mighty oil.

CHAPTER 3

Supplements

Creatine

Creatine dietary supplements was the reserve of bodybuilders and health clubnasium bunnies alike and that is probably what involves thoughts while you listen the word. But current research on the University of Australia have proven that it may additionally assist supercharge your intellectual overall performance, raise your IQ and enhance your mastering cappotential all on the equal time. This take a look at observed that once taking creatine, topics may want to keep extra records and carry out higher on a huge kind of obligations than earlier than supplementation.

This amino acid is produced to your liver, kidneys and pancreas, and is saved to your muscle tissues earlier than being used. However, sure stresses, accidents or nutritional alternatives can have an impact on the stages of creatine to your frame, adverse your overall performance and harming your mind electricity, so supplementing with it is probably the name of the game for more mind electricity which you are searching for.

You can get it in pill form; purpose for 5,000mg in line with day.

Omega-3 Fatty Acids

Omega-three fatty acids (DHA) are the kings of mind safety and reminiscence promotion, gambling a function withinside the improvement of the mind withinside the womb and assisting mind mobileular membranes talk efficaciously. It's advised that as much as 75% of the populace are poor on this critical fat, and that this deficiency may be contributing to all sorts of ailments such as depression, ADHD and Alzheimer's disease. Obviously, in case your mind signalling gadget isn't operating withinside the manner it's prepurported to then you'll be averted from focussing, questioning and appearing withinside the manner which you should.

Omega-three fatty acids have additionally proven to save you the buildup of mind plaque that could result in degenerative mind diseases, and additionally assist enhance your universal reminiscence in case you aren't a sufferer.

Great meals reassets consist of nuts, mainly walnuts, flaxseed, and additionally beans. In this case, wholefood reassets are advanced to supplementing. If you do pick to supplement, purpose for 1,two hundred to 2,400mg in line with day.

Anti-Oxidants

If you've study thru the preceding thirty herbal treatments that could raise your mind, you may absolute confidence recognize through now that antioxidants have a massive function to play, each withinside the safety of our brains from the ravages of age, however additionally protective them from infection and cognitive decline.

They consist of beta-carotene, lutein, lycopene, selenium, diet A, diet C and diet E, to call however some.

Their primary motion is certainly considered one among protective your complete frame from free-radical damage. Free-radicals are the dangerous materials which get up because the end result of oxidative pressure, along with environmental stresses, emotional pressure and different pollution which we would come upon. Whilst lots of those stressors are processed efficaciously through the frame, in this contemporary age we come upon a amount this is some distance better than ever visible earlier than. Just take pollution, alcoholism, demanding jobs, medicines and smoking as a few examples.

This is wherein antioxidants come in. They war those unfastened radicals which also can have an effect on our cognitive functioning and permit us to revel in higher reminiscence and a extra green thoughts all on the equal time.

Luckily, it's highly smooth to get all which you want in case you devour a numerous weight loss program, inclusive of as a minimum nine portions of fruit and greens each unmarried day. In truth, ingesting an ample plant-primarily based totally weight loss program is the only manner to acquire lots of antioxidants.

Alpha GPC (L-alpha-glycerylphosphorylcholine)

Alpha GPC is a awesome shape of choline that the frame can without difficulty use to construct your mind cells, accelerate your mastering, enhance your reminiscence and additionally improve your wondering power. This nootropic has visible a surge in recognition these days because of its capacity to pass the blood-mind barrier and improve your grey matter.

Choline is a B-complicated nutrition that is really a precursor of the crucial neurotransmitter acetylcholine. It is that this acetylcholine that allows the mind cells to speak effectively, and is likewise the neurotransmitter that decreases withinside the brains of Alzheimer's and dementia sufferers. Additionally, it protects the mind from nerve mobileular demise and harm and will really stimulate nerve cells to regenerate. It additionally works as a relaxing substance withinside the frame, supporting to lessen stages of strain and tension.

And similarly to all of this, research have proven that it may really boom dopamine concentrations withinside the mind, and assist you to experience extra encouraged and 'switched on' and supercharge your mastering and reminiscence.

The nice meals reassets of choline encompass soymilk, tofu, quinoa, and broccoli. However, in case you would love to assure your intake, select a complement instead.

To supply your self a modest improve, complement with 600mg according to day, or boom to round 1200mg in case you are tormented by cognitive issues inclusive of Alzheimer's.

Acetyl-l-Carnitine (ALC)

Acetyl-l-Carnitine (ALC) is a evidently going on amino acid which can enhance your temper and consciousness and in reality assist you to study faster. It works as an antioxidant to defend the tissues of your anxious machine and mind from unfastened-radical harm and sicknesses inclusive of Alzheimer's and dementia.

Your frame really produces its very own model of l-carnitine, however extra day by day supplementation would possibly simply supply your frame the improve that it needs. It works through boosting the mitochondrial interest withinside the cells of your frame, some thing this is specifically useful in terms of your mind. After all,
excessive stages of electricity withinside the mind cells interprets to higher and extra green notion tactics.

You can discover acetyl-l-carnitine (ALC) in positive foods, inclusive of avocados, *asparagus and whole-wheat bread,* and additionally to make certain which you are becoming sufficient nutrition C on your weight loss program to help your kidneys and liver and boom your very own production.

If you select to complement, choose among one thousand to 3000mg according to day.

5-HTP

The nice serotonin booster accessible available in the marketplace is 5-HTP, in truth it's been stated that it's miles natures nice and only shape of Prozac. It really comes from a West African tree named Griffonia simplicifolia and crosses the blood-mind barrier without difficulty earlier than being transformed to a sort of serotonin. So in case you need to raise your temper and your reminiscence, flip to 5-HTP.

As you could remember, serotonin is concerned with many crucial tactics withinside the frame, and coffee stages of it may make a contribution to low temper, depression, tension and insomnia. When you improve those stages, you'll now no longer simplest assist your self experience higher, however you'll be capable of carry that intellectual fog that frequently stands among you and remembering all the data which you want to.

You can't get 5-HTP from meals, however you may without difficulty discover it as a complement- take round three hundred to 500mg according to day. It works nice with St John's Wort as each herbs paintings synergistically. Do now no longer take 5-HTP or St John's Wort in case you are taking antidepressant medications - first discuss with your doctor.

Co Enzyme Q-10

Co Enzyme Q10 is a evidently going on substance that allows us to provide electricity withinside the cells of our our bodies and works as an antioxidant to defend mobileular membranes and DNA from unfastened-radical harm. Better than that, it'd really assist to opposite the ageing manner and upload round 9 more years to our lives. Sounds awesome, doesn't it?

Co Enzyme Q10 works through repairing mitochondria, and supporting them to go back to their authentic state. Mitochondria are observed at some point of the human frame, suggesting that if the cells for your frame are greater youthful, so can be your mind cells. The apparent end is higher wondering and learning.

It may assist to put off the onset of age-associated reminiscence loss and dementia, Alzheimer's disorder and additionally Parkinson's, making it one of the pleasant all-spherical dietary supplements out there.

If you'd want to experience the blessings for yourself, complement with doses of among three hundred and 1,200mg in line with day.

Vitamins B6, B12 and Folic Acid

All B-complicated nutrients are critical for life, making sure our mind and worried system's boom and improvement and supporting us to extract the vitamins from our meals and use it in our cells. These include:

- B1 (thiamine)

- B2 (Riboflavin)

- B3 (Niacin)

- B5 (Pantothenic Acid)

- B6 (Pyridoxine)

- B7 (Biotin)

- B9 (Folic acid)

- B12 (cobalamin)

It's critical to get our day by day dose of all of them, as they're water-soluble and the frame is not able to save any excess. This method that deficiency can pretty without problems occur, particularly if we aren't paying our traditional interest to our diets.
This is particularly the case with B6, B12 and Folic acid. In fact, people with decrease B12 and folic acid degrees of their blood are much more likely to increase Alzheimer's disorder.

Studies have proven that supplementing with all 3 of those assist to stave off Alzheimer's, as they decrease degrees of homocysteine withinside the frame, that's related to shrinkage to the mind.

So make certain you have become an ok nutritional consumption of all the B- complicated nutrients, particularly the 'magic 3'. Folic acid is simple to discover in all forms of inexperienced leafy veggies, beans, orange juice, dried peas and citrus fruit. B6 may be observed in culmination and vegetables, particularly bananas, and at the same time as B12 is tougher to discover in plant foods, it could be observed in brewer's yeast and different fortified products. You can, of course, take a complement to make certain all of those nutrients were taken care of.

Vitamin D

Vitamin D is absolutely a hormone this is synthesised whilst daylight hits your pores and skin. Adequate degrees of the stuff assist you to experience tremendous and energized and preserve wholesome hearts and bones. The problem is that too many humans put on sunscreen on day by day basis, or cowl themselves totally with apparel in order that the solar doesn't absolutely contact their pores and skin at all. Or they may even stay in northern regions that revel in a loss of daylight at some point of a great share of the year. This is whilst supplementation turns into essential.

Vitamin D stimulates degrees of the hormone serotonin, which lifts our moods and makes us experience right approximately ourselves. You see, there truely is a motive why we experience uplifted on a sunny, cloudless day.

So attempt to get out withinside the daylight every time feasible for brief time period to experience the uplifting blessings. You also can take a complement in case you stay in a chillier climate - round 15 micrograms (or six hundred UI) in line with day is ideal. Your healthcare practitioner may also advise you are taking greater in case you discover you're diet D deficient.

High-Quality Multivitamin And Mineral

Diet performs a large position in keeping the fitness of your mind and making sure you experience incredible and carry out at the very best stage feasible. The vitamins that your meals comprise assist help mind processes, manipulate hormonal degrees and

actually feed your mind, developing new mind cells and constructing communication.

Certain nutrients and minerals which include B-complicated nutrients, magnesium, manganese, diet D, beta carotene, diet C and diet E are particularly essential in terms of minimizing the outcomes of oxidation and save you the onset of Alzheimer's, reminiscence loss and dementia.

But every so often we don't deliver our diets our complete interest, or we accidently go away gaps withinside the vitamins we have become thru lack of know-how or forgetfulness. It's now no longer usually smooth to cowl all your bases, and that's whilst taking a multivitamin and mineral complement can assist.

So my final tip for you need to be to take a excessive exceptional diet and mineral complement that consists of the whole lot you need, is made through a depended on logo and is low cost for you too.

CHAPTER 4

Super Foods & Lifestyle

Beautiful Berries

There's not anything pretty like tucking right into a large bowl of freshly picked berries. Blueberries, strawberries, raspberries, loganberries - they're all completely delicious.

And they're all brilliant to your intellectual overall performance too.

It's generally assumed that that is because of the tremendous amount of antioxidants that they incorporate. These save you the body's cells from harm via way of means of free-radicals and assist save you the formation of plaque round mind tissues, that's one of the foremost reasons of Alzheimer's disease.

But in fact, that is simplest a part of the story. An article in The Journal of Agricultural and Food Chemistry mentioned that they assist enhance signalling withinside the mind, and assist lessen inflammation, which improves motor characteristic and boosts wondering electricity. They're additionally packed complete of vitamins inclusive of diet K, diet C, manganese and copper.

All berries also are packed complete of a compound referred to as anthocyanin, that's what offers them their wealthy darkish colour and works as an powerful anti- inflammatory for the entire body.

Experts suggest that we must be treating ourselves to round 3 quantities of berries each unmarried week. Sounds like it's approximately time to take pleasure in a scrumptious super-meals berry smoothie!

Nutritious Nuts

The absolute quality manner to get sufficient mind-constructing omega-three fatty acids in our diets is to nibble on a handful of nuts each day.

Not simplest are they scrumptious, filling and packed complete of important nutrients and minerals inclusive of diet E, *iron, zinc and magnesium,* in addition they incorporate sizeable quantities of DHA, a kind of omega-three that improves cognitive performance, upkeep age-associated reminiscence harm or even boosts the brains of new-born infants and facilitates relieve signs of ADHA in kids. Phew- what a mouthful!

Nuts additionally incorporate excessive stages of the B-nutrients, that are turning into more and more more tough to eat withinside the present day diet, and additionally assist help your apprehensive system, construct new cells and sell intellectual fitness.

If you're having problem selecting I'd recommend you choose walnuts. They truely are the quality of the bunch as they postpone mind getting old and increase mind- electricity in a single hit. Almonds also are tremendous for grey remember because of their excessive stages of diet E, and are truely flexible and yummy - however any will make a large distinction for your mind-electricity.

Enjoy a small handful each day (and no, you shouldn't fear approximately the calories!)

Awesome Avocados

Avocados are one of these meals which can be underrated, and in reality till some years ago, a few fitness figures encouraged to live farfar from them because of their fats content material.

That is, till they located that this fats content material turned into tremendous at assisting to push back dementia and mind getting old, in addition to boosting your general fitness.
This fats is referred to as oleic acid and facilitates to construct myelin in our brains, and permits our concept tactics to end up greater efficient. Sounds good, doesn't it?

It's stated that avocados are most of the maximum whole meals at the planet, and what's now no longer to love approximately them? They're wealthy, they're creamy and that they supply an general increase to some thing meal you may ever dream up.

They're additionally packed complete of nutrients and minerals, excessive in protein and additionally
assist increase the stages of a neurotransmitter referred to as dopamine on your body, assisting you sense greater targeted and happy.

Avocados may be eaten in such a lot of ways, however my absolute favored needs to be in a scrumptious, colourful salad. Aim to eat round 1/2 of an avocado each couple of days.

Cocoa For Creativity

Great information for each chocolate-lover out there - cocoa lets you sense good, don't forget greater of what you're mastering and to attention like a ninja!

But the reality is, the advantages rely on the nice of the chocolate and the manner you pick out to eat it. I'm afraid plucking a family-sized bar off the cabinets of your neighborhood shop isn't going to be excuse sufficient - you want it darkish, natural and dairy-free.

Cocoa works miracles on our brains due to the fact it's excessive in styles of compounds that sell a wholesome mind - those are flavonoids and flavanols. Flavonoids are a kind of antioxidant that enhance reminiscence, attention and interest and assist to clean out detrimental free-radicals from the cells of our bodies. Flavanols are a particular kind of flavonoid, which facilitates to enhance blood float to the mind for round to a few hours after consumption.

Let's now no longer overlook that cocoa additionally incorporates excessive stages of the mineral magnesium, which additionally facilitates to sell reminiscence and mastering, in addition to having a calming impact upon the entire body. Sounds like a incredible excuse to devour greater!

The final manner to experience cocoa is to buy a few natural and unadulterated uncooked cacao electricity and upload it for your baked goods, smoothies and desserts.
Unfortunately there isn't an RDA of cocoa so it's as much as you to locate the satisfactory dosage for you - a bit is going an extended manner.

Green Tea

Green tea. Love it or hate it? Most folks have attempted its barely sour and earthy taste for ourselves, however in case you haven't you need to truely supply it a pass. As some distance as liquids pass, it's approximately as wholesome because it gets. Not simplest does it incorporate superb quantities of polyphenols, the antioxidants that assist defend our our bodies and brains from the harm of unfastened radicals; it's additionally excessive in an amino acid known as l-theanine which promotes exquisite mood, getting to know and reminiscence. And the advantages don't simply prevent there.

Studies achieved through the University of Basel, Switzerland have located that inexperienced tea improves your intellectual overall performance and reminiscence, supporting to enhance age-associated reminiscence decline. Along with the plaque-lowering impact it has upon the mind, inexperienced tea may be an appropriate technique to assist defy dementia and Alzheimer's disorder too.

In some other take a look at supplied on the 2015 International Conference on Alzheimer's and Parkinson's Diseases, counseled that inexperienced tea intake turned into connected to much less intellectual decline, whether or not this turned into a every day dose, a weekly dose, or someplace in between.

Green tea additionally carries a substantial quantity of caffeine, which allows to enhance your cognizance and your intellectual overall performance. In truth it sincerely carries round 24mg of caffeine in each cup, as compared to round 14mg in a cup of black tea and round 47mg in an espresso, so don't pass overboard at the stuff. Black tea additionally stocks comparable advantages as inexperienced tea, so pick out the only you revel in the most.

Aim to drink at the least one cup of inexperienced or black tea in line with week, or greater in case you truly revel in the taste. If you're now no longer a fan, you could additionally locate inexperienced tea drugs at your nearest fitness meals store.

Broccoli

Broccoli is one of the actual super-ingredients that has stood the check of time and is surely splendid on your mind and your overall performance, similarly to the relaxation of your frame. This is due to the fact it's excessive in a substance referred to as lignans. This is a phytoestrogen this is concerned with most efficient questioning consisting of reasoning and remembering.

It's additionally a exquisite manner of shielding your frame from primary apprehensive system

decline, consisting of the sort visible in Alzheimer's disorder. As located through researchers at King's College, London, broccoli carries excessive degrees of a compound known as glucosinates, which inhibit the movement of a neuron-unfavourable enzyme known as acetylcholinesterase, which can be connected to the onset of the disorder.

And similarly to all of that, broccoli is likewise a exquisite supply of a B-complicated nutrition known as choline, which sincerely boosts degrees of the important thing neurotransmitter acetylcholine. This allows enhance cognitive function, promotes intellectual readability and allows you broaden a higher short-time period reminiscence than you ever concept possible.

Enjoy broccoli numerous instances in line with week as a part of your meal or a yummy side- dish.

Beets

Beets assist you to revel in greater energy, each mentally and physically. This is due to the fact they incorporate beneficiant quantities of herbal nitrates which, whilst eaten, get transformed to nitric oxide. This permits the partitions of your blood vessels to expand, together with the ones on your mind so that you get that greater increase of oxygen and energy. As you could imagine, this takes your cognitive overall performance to an entire new level.

They also are the simplest supply of the phytonutrients known as betalains. These have an anti-oxidant and anti inflammatory impact upon the mind and the frame, and can even assist to address cancers and age-associated decline.

Be conscious that those betalains are instead unstable, so for satisfactory effects, revel in your beets juiced or simplest gently cooked. I love grating sparkling beets right into a salad or including them to a sparkling juice. And of course, your urine might also broaden a barely purple tinge after ingesting beets, however that's not anything you want to fear approximately.

Spinach

Your dad and mom had been proper once they informed you to consume up your greens! Just one serving in line with day of spinach, spring greens, kale or collards packs a dietary punch and could assist lessen cognitive decline and reminiscence loss.

It's packed complete of critical minerals that may be tough to get from different meals sources, and is excessive withinside the antioxidant, lutein, which allows to sell effecting getting to know, language and reminiscence.

Researchers at Rush University in Chicago additionally determined that people who consume a each day serving of vegetables have brains which can be round eleven years more youthful than their organic age. They advise that this is probably thanks to the excessive ranges of diet K. Vitamin K is a nutrient of special interest in the field of brain medicine as it plays an important role in blood clotting and regulating the amount of calcium in the brain - both benefits that can improve the symptoms experienced by Alzheimer's sufferers.

You can experience all of those blessings through consuming a number of inexperienced leafy veggies, now no longer simply spinach. Why now no longer upload a each day part of brussel sprouts, kale, collards, Swiss chard, cauliflower or maybe cabbage on your weight loss program to achieve a few high-quality effects.

Water

I understand what you're questioning - water isn't even a meals! And you're clearly right, however much like meals it's one of the primary basics of existence and merits a mention.

Our brains are round 85% water, and depend upon this water to offer the electric electricity for concept procedures and cognition to occur. Therefore it makes a ton of feel that in case you overlook about to drink sufficient water, you threat unfavourable your energy of cognition, studying cappotential and additionally temper withinside the process. Dehydration is likewise related intently to dementia, Alzheimer's disease, Parkinson's, Autism or even ADHD. Studies have proven that only a 1% drop in hydration effects in a 5% lower in performance. Do the mathsematics and you may see how critical it's miles to hold hydrated!

And now no longer most effective that, one take a look at determined that scholars who took a bottle of water into an examination truly done higher and were given higher grades than the ones that didn't.

It's all too smooth to neglect about approximately consuming sufficient water, specifically if we've busy lives. We wait till we sense thirst and surprise why it doesn't appear to assist. Thirst is a past due signal of dehydration and you may in all likelihood sense the consequences earlier than you truly sense like a drink.

So make certain you drink water regularly, whether or not you sense thirsty or now no longer. Invest in a reusable aluminium bottle and sip during the day. Aim to drink among 2-three liters for max hydration and surest performance.

Garlic

Garlic offers such a lot of blessings on your health, you'd be clearly stupid now no longer to get your each day dose, and it's a real super-meals on the subject of enhancing your temper, reminiscence and focus (in addition to a number of different things).

It incorporates a rich of sulphuric compounds that own excellent anti-oxidant homes and may tackle nearly any infection you can suppose of. One of those, referred to as FruArg is specially thrilling to us as it performs a shielding position on mind cells, supporting them to face up to life-style stresses like consuming an excessive amount of alcohol, smoking, maintaining a mind harm and persistent strain.

Garlic additionally promotes higher blood go with the drift to the whole frame, together with the mind, and has been proven to combat sure cancers while studied in lab conditions.
Lastly, garlic will assist enhance your reminiscence, your temper and your studying through growing the ranges of 5-hydroxytryptamine (5-HTP) ranges for your mind. This is a form of serotonin receptor, with the intention to assist you sense great, enhance your motivation, assist you to experience greater rejuvenating sleep AND recollect the whole lot you want to less difficult than earlier than than.

Garlic is scrumptious and clearly easy to feature on your ordinary weight loss program. If you're now no longer a fan, choose garlic tablets or capsules instead. You can ingest among three hundred to 1,000mg of garlic extract in line with day, relying for your wishes.

Think Positively

The idea which you should 'suppose greater positively' may come off as sounding barely strange, however there's an entire heap of studies to show that it truly does paintings wonders on the subject of feeling happier and greater fantastic approximately your existence; like taking part in readability of concept, shielding your self from age-associated reminiscence loss and heightening your intellectual performance.

The motives are clear. The maximum influential a part of our lives isn't how tons cash we've withinside the bank, nor how knowledgeable we are, nor what form of process we would have. It's truly how we see the arena, in different words, our perspective. If you spot the arena as a threatening location and consider which you aren't worth to say your very own position inside it, your frame will react as though it have been true, the ranges of strain hormones for your frame will skyrocket and your questioning becomes clumsy and clouded. As a end result you'll age quicker and sense unhappier.

But in case you rather give attention to the effective things, downplaying the awful and feeling gratitude for the suitable, then you'll permit your self to blossom, lessen degrees of strain hormones and growth degrees of the satisfied hormones too.

This doesn't suggest pretending that the whole lot is first-rate while deep down you already know that it isn't, however it does suggest taking the time to look what's lovely to your existence. It all begins offevolved proper there with you.

Get Moving

Humans have been by no means designed to stay the styles of sedentary lives that we do today. We take a seat down to devour breakfast, we climb into the automobile and take a seat down as we shuttle to work, we take a seat down all day at our desks running tough on our computer systems and we repeat the technique while we arrive home, feeling so exhausted that we come to a decision the sofa for the relaxation of the evening. This loss of motion is what's killing our brains and our intelligence slowly.

For our brains and our bodies to characteristic as they should, we want to transport our our bodies, we want to get blood flowing thru our cerebral blood vessels and pour crucial oxygen into our mind cells. We want the stimulation of the sparkling air

for our senses and to experience the wholesome endorphins flood our system.

The most effective manner to do that is to get extra exercise. Now, don't panic, I don't always suggest sweating it out withinside the nearest gym (even though that wouldn't be a awful idea!).

Instead, start with the aid of using welcoming motion into your existence. Take the steps in preference to the lift, park in addition away and stroll the few final blocks to work, rise up out of your table each hour and take a toilet break, head out and feature a walk withinside the sparkling air. It all counts.

You may even down load an app on your phone in case you want assist with this. A suitable vicinity to begin is with a pedometer app, which counts your paces and lets you attain the perfect 10,000 steps in step with day. What ought to you do to attain this target?

Quit Processed and Artificial Sweeteners

If you've got got study my book, *Healthy Living: 30 Powerful Daily Habits,* you'll have visible the blessings that quitting processed and synthetic sweeteners may have upon your fitness as a complete. Right now we're going to give attention to the damage this stuff do on your mind.

Now, it's generally sugar that receives the awful press, being deemed as a 'white poison', and even as that is true, it's most effective a part of the story. When human beings pay attention that sugar is detrimental to their fitness, they regularly flip to synthetic sweeteners rather, wondering that they're appearing a kindness to their frame and supporting themselves to heal. What they don't realize is that synthetic sweeteners may truly be worse for you than sugar.

The synthetic sweetener this is used maximum broadly in weight loss plan gentle beverages and ingredients is aspartame. Studies have demonstrated a sturdy hyperlink among this synthetic chemical and mind damage. That's proper - aspartame ought to truly be harming your mind-strength, affecting your idea procedures and in the end making you stupider.

So what do you devour when you have a candy teeth however need to shield

your mind? The maximum healthy manner to get a bit sweetness into your existence is to revel in complete ingredients including fruit, which now no longer most effective have that high-quality flavor you so
crave, however additionally offer a mess of mind-boosting vitamins and antioxidants.

Become Bilingual

Want to reinforce your mind-strength and language-processing skills, in addition to put off the viable onset of Alzheimer's and dementia? Experts endorse that being bilingual can assist to gradual age-associated mind decline and develop new mind connections. But you don't need to be older to revel in its blessings. One observe confirmed that teens who spoke a couple of language outperformed their monolingual peers.

Let's delve a bit deeper to recognize why. For a monolingual person, the use of language will most effective ever prompt one facet of the mind. However, for the bilinguals, each aspects of the mind are energetic while the use of language. This approach that a mind this is extra comprehensively 'exercised' and healthier as a result, now no longer simply with regards to languages.

And because the icing at the cake, researchers on the University of Ghent observed that bilingualism can put off the onset of Alzheimer's with the aid of using round 4 years. Sounds like it's time to dig out the ones vintage textbooks!

Get Your Sleep

Life's too brief to waste hours sleeping, proper? Actually, that's twisted logic. Getting sufficient sleep is the very best and best manner to reinforce your mind-strength and experience lively and revived the subsequent day. And higher still, it doesn't fee a cent and could make you experience terrific too.

When we sleep, we deliver our our bodies the threat to recharge, each bodily and mentally. We deliver it the possibility to clean out the informational enter we were supplying it over the direction of the day, maintain what is right and trash what isn't. In a nutshell, sleep allows us examine and preserve greater information.

We all understand what it's like while you are sleep-deprived. Your mind feels foggy, you're grumpy and irritable, you emerge as forgetful, clumsy and the entirety looks as if an massive effort. If you start to prioritize sleep, all of this could emerge as a factor of the beyond and you'll experience prepared to address what lifestyles may throw at you.

So do it! From this very moment, vow to position your frame first and make sleep a concern to peer a few extremely good results. Experts advocate which you need to get round 8 hours of sleep in line with night, however the proper determine clearly does rely upon the individual - I locate that a determine in the direction of 9 works first-class with me, however locate what works first-class for you.

Listen To Music

Not simplest is track a exquisite deal with that assist you to experience uplifted, alive and happy, it may additionally have a few clearly brilliant advantages for you memory, awareness and interest, language talents AND bodily coordination. Sounds like a brilliant cause to position on a number of your favourite tunes, in case you ask me!

It works with the aid of using activating each facets of your mind, sporting activities each a part of it, and will increase the interest withinside the corpus callosum - the relationship among each facets of your mind. In addition, it additionally has an impact upon our feelings and lets in us to transport to an area past language. This TED animation by Anita Collins explains what happens in the brain when you play a musical instrument, however is likewise beneficial in relation to knowledge the impact that track has upon the mind. Take a look.

The take-domestic message is to simply 'pay attention to greater track'. Rediscover your favourite tracks, transfer off the tv and permit track wake up your mind and your senses.

Avoid Monosodium Glutamate (MSG)

MSG, or monosodium glutamate is a meals additive that works as a taste enhancer and is mechanically brought to many Asian ingredients and canned goods. The awful information is that it acts as a neurotoxin (and destroys mind cells and as a

result), negatively impacts mind characteristic and reasons a extensive variety of signs including headaches, dizziness, diarrhoea, excessive blood pressure, excessive blood sugar tiers and additionally imaginative and prescient damage.

It works with the aid of using hyper-stimulating the nerves and approaches withinside the whole frame as much as the factor of damage. There are severa research that guide this fact, including the only accomplished on the Robert S. Dow Neurobiology Laboratories in Portland, which observed that MSG reasons neuron demise and associated conditions.

The problem with MSG is that it isn't always mechanically labelled so it may be hard to understand while you is probably ingesting it, or not. The first-class direction of movement is to keep away from processed elements which you can not pronounce, and rather give attention to consuming nutritious, sparkling wholefoods to be able to feed your frame and your mind.

Meditate

Imagine if you can enhance your mind with the aid of using doing 'nothing'? Does that sound too suitable to be proper? You'll be thrilled to understand that that is nearly sure in case you select to absorb a mediation practice. You'll experience more potent and happier, much less pressured and greater centered at the matters in lifestyles that clearly count to you.

If you've got got ever experimented with mediation withinside the beyond, you'll understand that when a session, regardless of how short, you experience energized and uplifted and additionally at peace with the world. These emotions you would possibly have skilled have additionally been backed-up with bloodless tough technological know-how too.

Meditation has been validated to paintings higher than prescribed drugs for depression, improves tiers of awareness and concentration, protects the growing old mind with the aid of using growing the quantity and density of your grey count, and decreases tension too.

It's quite simple to begin mediating. Just discover a quiet region and permit your interest to observe the movement of your breath. And this is nearly all there's to it. If you're having problem locating the time to practice, begin with only some mins each day. There are many 30-day mediation demanding situations obtainable that may assist come up with the frenzy you want to begin.

Practice Yoga

Yoga is the time-examined technique of locating internal peace and outer energy on the identical time. Its advantages consist of decreasing stress, assisting you to sleep, enhancing your mood, assisting you aleven though grief, recovery low self- esteem issues, and additionally assisting you experience brilliant.

It works in plenty the equal manner as meditation with the aid of using encouraging you to consciousness at the breath, however not like mediation, yoga encourages you to apply your frame as you do so. It's an exquisite manner to locate internal power and consciousness and placed you again in contact together along with your frame and your internal world. All of these items frequently receives buried underneath the insanity of cutting-edge life, so it could be very recuperation to locate it again.

It also can paintings wonders for melancholy and assist stimulate your consciousness and your facts retention. So in place of hitting the caffeine earlier than an critical exam, why now no longer take a yoga magnificence instead?

HABIT 1
Eat Plants

Plants create life. Plants promote incredible health, energy and longevity. Plants are absolutely amazing.

They're packed complete of the nutrients and minerals that your frame craves for maximum fitness, and provide beneficiant portions of most cancers-preventing antioxidants and crucial fiber with a view to hold your intestine running great. The excellent and only manner to experience more fit and more potent is to experience an ample amount of clean culmination and vegetables. And of course, in case you're seeking to lessen your waistline you'll be thrilled to pay attention that culmination and vegetables are excessive in vitamins even as low in calories, and genuinely scrumptious - so, *consume up!*

But of course, you understand all of this, don't you? You'd had been residing on Mars for the beyond few many years to have ignored this crucial facts. Yet come what may alongside the manner, we will all succumb to temptations, fall off the wagon, and slip into bad habits, filling our diets with bad processed meals and fitness-negative portions of saturated fats.

As nicely as growing your intake of plants, I'd additionally urge you to lessen animal merchandise out of your eating regimen, consisting of meat, fish, eggs, milk and different dairy merchandise, and choose healthier, plant-primarily based totally options consisting of non-dairy milk (almond, *coconut or rice milks, for example),* beneficiant every day servings of whole-grains (gluten loose in case you are intolerant), hearty and healthy root vegetables, and protein-wealthy legumes, nuts and seeds. Although we understand animal merchandise to be a wholeSome supply of protein, as compared to plant reassets they may be more difficult to digest, excessive in saturated fats, worsen fitness situations consisting of eczema, acne, bronchial allergies and arthritis, and might make contributions to greater extreme long-time period situations consisting of diabetes and coronary heart sickness. So, why now no longer experience fantastic fitness with the aid of using absolutely changing those 'dead' meals with energy-wealthy, nutrient wealthy, *stay plants?*

Challenge yourself to eat a plant-rich diet for 30 days. You'll be amazed to see your energy levels increase and the pounds melt away.

It's awesome clean to get started. Simply fill your plate with as many vegetables,
legumes and whole-grains as you could and experience. Then in place of ingesting fitness-negative cakes, cookies and ice creams, experience a scrumptious fruit smoothie or colourful fruit salad to spherical off your meal.

You also can upload more vegetables into any recipe which you are cooking to enhance your vitamins, specially cruciferous ones like broccoli, cauliflower or for even greater fitness-boosting effects, masses of inexperienced leafy vegetables. *By making those easy changes, your frame will thank you!*

HABIT 2

Opt for Wholefood Fats

We need to be paying greater attention to getting the *right* kinds of fats, in their natural forms and eaten as part of a wholefood diet.

The hassle with a few low-fats diets is that even as human beings consciousness closely on simply the amount of fats they may be ingesting, they forget to consider crucial things; the sort of fat they consume and the country in their eating regimen as a whole.

Now first permit me come up with an critical fact - our our bodies want a few fats to function. Our brains are in large part composed of fats and we want to consume 'appropriate fat' to offer us with energy, hold a wholesome apprehensive system, hold pores and skin and cells wholesome, to hold the fats-primarily based totally nutrients A, D and E, and to assist adjust our hormonal processes. This isn't always to mention we need to consume fat in excess, though. Balance is key, and what we want to be specializing in is ditching the awful fat and changing them with the best.

What are the best and awful fat? In a nutshell, appropriate fat are those of their herbal paperwork which are contained inside wholefoods consisting of avocados, almonds, olives, coconuts, walnuts and chia seeds.

The awful fat are those which are rather processed, of animal starting place and refill all of these junk meals, speedy meals and prepackaged meals that many human beings want to consume.
These styles of fat come below principal categories: *saturated fat and trans fat which could growth your chance of coronary heart sickness and cholesterol*, reason obesity, growth your dangers of diabetes, make contributions to most cancers and lots of different fitness situations.

For a long term now, monounsaturated and polyunsaturated fat had been taken into consideration to be the more healthy ones, being excessive in omega-3's and forming a part of the well-known Mediterranean weight loss program. This is, however, handiest a part of the story.
Let's now no longer overlook that oils are processed, low in vitamins while thinking about their excessive calorie content, and in the end fattening meals that need to be decreased via way of means of anybody with premier fitness in sight.

It's a long way higher to revel in a crunchy and pleasant handful of nuts and seeds and get a first-rate dose of heart-defensive vitamins withinside the manner nature intended, rather than frying your falafel in a bucket of oil or drenching your salad leaves with the stuff and seeking to claim it healthful.

By following a plant-wealthy weight loss program with masses of entire meals, simply because the Mediterranean's do, while fending off the processed stuff as a good deal as possible, you'll be properly for your manner to getting the pleasant sort of healthful fat that your frame needs.

HABIT 3
Clear Out the Junk

You realize what it's like. You begin with handiest the pleasant of intentions: you'll persist with healthful meals, and you'll keep away from nasty additives, preservatives, poisonous processed fat and sugars. Of route you'll. Because you're an knowledgeable man or woman and you've invested it slow into coming across what works pleasant to your frame, and as a end result you've vowed to make the ones sorts of lasting modifications so that it will defend your frame, raise your energy, narrow your waistline and come up with that glow!

The problem is, you've simply arrived domestic after a specifically attempting day and you're seeking out some thing to cheer you up and praise your self with. So you open up the fridge or cupboard and pull out the ones large luggage of potato chips, double chocolate cookies or own circle of relatives-sized packs of sweet and dive proper on in, hoping to locate solace withinside the backside in their fats and sugar-weighted down pack.

But does it ever work? Do you *really* feel better after you've stuffed in enough junk to feed a party of people?

The solution is a huge and resounding 'no!'

What you turn out to be feeling is guilt and anger; anger with your self for tossing away your fitness for the sake of a whim, and guilt which you have eaten on this grasping and unfavourable manner.

So what are you able to do to prevent all of this going on withinside the first place? You in reality clean the junk meals out of your domestic (and your desk, your car, or your handbag for that matter). It's quite logical, isn't it? If it's now no longer there, you can't consume it. Cravings of this kind are commonly whimsical and opportunistic in nature, and if you're fuelled up at the proper meals, you're not likely to locate your self riding the thirty mins to the shop simply to get that processed sugar repair which you don't truly want.

Don't ever allow junk meals into your domestic, now no longer even in case your children beg you desperately or your companion complains. Instead throw away or donate the ones tempting meals and fill your cabinets with more healthy options and

wholefood goodness. Why now no longer inventory up on butter-unfastened popcorn for a touch crunch, or pleasant, wholegrain crackers with sparkling tomato and home made hummus dip? You'll be doing you and your own circle of relatives a huge choose and making sure which you all revel in longer and more healthy lives, with trimmer waistlines as a end result!

HABIT 4
Enjoy Fermented Foods

A buddy of mine become continually notably supportive and inspiring after I endeavored on my adventure to higher fitness. But of route I'd assume her to be
- she'd been a veggie munching, yoga-working towards pioneer of simplicity for years. But as quickly as she commenced making a song the praises of strange-sounds meals like kimchi, sauerkraut, kombucha and kefir, I couldn't assist however increase my eyebrows and byskip these items off as 'crunchy' meals. That is, till I skilled the blessings for myself.

As you may already realize approximately me from my Healthy Gut Solution book, I'd been laid low with digestive troubles that I simply couldn't shake off for years
- whether or not it become bloating, indigestion, diarrhea, trapped wind or cramps, you can assure that I'd be afflicted by some thing. I'd attempted all sorts of matters over the years, from peppermint capsules, to teas to wheat luggage and all sorts of different matters. But it become handiest after I wiped clean up my weight loss program and integrated those fermented meals that I truly observed a difference.

So what are fermented foods and how can they help?

Fermentation is a conventional manner of retaining meals with out the want for vacuum packs, canning or the usage of stupid quantities of chemical preservatives.

The method works with the aid of using the usage of yeast or micro organism, which converts the sugars gift into alcohol. The end result is a meals this is simpler to digest, better in important nutrients and omega-3's, and additionally excessive in digestive enzymes. It additionally will increase the quantity of healthful micro organism to your intestine, which improves your digestion, eases signs and symptoms of IBS, acne, arthritis, despair or even persistent migraine. You'd be silly now no longer to consist of a few to your weight loss plan.

Why now no longer attempt a few kimchi, sauerkraut, kombucha or kefir and spot which one you like the quality? You could make all of them very inexpensively at domestic with out the want to go to the fitness meals store, making it price range pleasant in addition to fitness- pleasant.

Take a look at my _Healthy Gut Solution_ book if you'd like further statistics on intestine fitness and the way to enhance it.

HABIT 5
Say Goodbye to Processed & Artificial Sweeteners

We experience sugar due to the fact we've been programmed to for survival, a trick which served us nicely till we hit the current age of over processing and we started out to strip ingredients away to inside an inch in their lives. These new 'naked' ingredients are without vitamins and intestine-pleasant fiber, and actually offer empty calories, that can depart our our bodies stressed and overworked. This is specially the case with white, subtle sugar and synthetic sweeteners.

An extra of subtle sugar at the side of a weight loss plan excessive in saturated fats is the wrongdoer in the back of such a lot of exclusive fitness situations consisting of inflammatory diseases, kind 2 diabetes, cancers, obesity, migraines, hormonal imbalance and people chronic cravings which you simply can't control.

And do not count on you're out of the woods in case you select synthetic chemical sweeteners to get your restore instead. The reality is, you are truely doing all of your frame greater damage than true with the aid of using deciding on them. Aspartame, that is one of the maximum broadly selected sweeteners and unearths its manner into weight loss plan sodas, low sugar ingredients or even gum, has been verified to be cancer-causing, can truely stimulate fats garage to your frame and aggravates an entire host of nasty fitness troubles.

What Can I Enjoy Instead?

So what alternatives do you've got got in case you nevertheless like a bit sweetness to your existence however are casting off processed sugars? Do you need to give up sugar altogether or is there a more healthy option? Let's locate out.

The quality manner to experience sweetness to your weight loss plan is with the aid of using eating wholefoods together with fruit. They offer the whole thing that nature supposed and feature a strong effect upon our blood sugar tiers due to the vitamins, water and fiber they comprise. They preserve our flavor buds satisfied and offer us with easy power even as taking higher care of our our bodies.

But in case you definitely do want that little some thing to feature for your natural tea or

bowl of oatmeal and fruit simply won't hit the spot, attempt greater herbal sweeteners together with coconut nectar, coconut sugar, natural maple syrup or stevia instead.

HABIT 6
Feed Your Mind with Mood-Boosting Foods

A simple way to help reach your happiness potential is to regularly consume 'mood-boosting' foods.

Low temper and despair can frequently be the end result of low tiers of a neurotransmitter known as serotonin, that is used for temper regulation, sexual choice and function, regulating our appetites, assisting us to sleep, boosting our reminiscence and getting to know abilities, regulating our temperatures and is even utilized in regulating our social behavior.

By consuming the proper varieties of meals, we will increase the tiers of serotonin in our our bodies and so correctly address temper-associated troubles with out resorting to pharmaceuticals with the nasty facet effects!

Whilst ingredients themselves don't truely comprise serotonin, many do comprise an amino acid known as tryptophan, which the frame can use to growth tiers of serotonin withinside the frame whilst eaten with carbohydrates. Luckily this amino acid is discovered abundantly in lots of culmination and greens that comprise protein, iron, nutrition B $_2$ and additionally nutrition B $_6$ - together with uncooked nuts (specially walnuts), *plantains, pineapples, bananas, kiwis, plums, tomatoes and tofu*, to call only a few.

Include greater of those ingredients to your weight loss plan and you may experience brighter, happier, greater active and stronger. Sounds true, doesn't it?

HABIT 7
Eat Enough

We were taught to take heed to consuming too much, however little can we ask ourselves, 'am I consuming enough?'

Perhaps you're dwelling a busy existence and frequently bypass food with out definitely that means to. Perhaps you experience which you can't squeeze withinside the time to stand up out of your table and seize a chew to eat. Perhaps you're so targeted with the project in hand which you don't experience the starvation pains after they arrive. Or possibly you're closely proscribing your consumption of nutritious ingredients withinside the attempt to lose weight.

Whatever your motives are, this dependancy is negatively affecting your productivity, killing your temper and depleting your strength tiers. Food is the gasoline that feeds our our bodies and minds to hold you working at your satisfactory. So in case you virtually do need to stay a more healthy and happier life, you should repair this dependancy earlier than your fitness starts offevolved to go through over time.

So, begin the perfect dependancy of all of them and revel in consuming healthfully in
abundance!

Make a vow to your self to prioritize consuming sufficient healthful energy till you're absolutely happy and satiated. Don't pass breakfast or lunch withinside the wish that it's going to assist you lose the ones more pounds (it won't paintings), and don't clutch a bag of chips or chocolate bar and suppose that's sufficient to hold you going. *It won't be.*

Instead, make the effort to disconnect and recharge your frame whilst you're nourishing your self. Take a healthful lunch with you to paintings, take a seat down and communicate together along with your own circle of relatives on the dinner desk as opposed to dashing to easy up, and ensure you continually have healthful snacks to your handbag or bag to hold you energized for success.

HABIT 8
Keep Hydrated

How much water do you drink over the course of an average day?

It's likely a bargain much less than you suppose.

Our our bodies are made up of fifty to 70% water, and we lose over 2.five liters of water every day thru perspiring, respiration and urinating. Replenishing our hydration is truely important for the right feature of each organ in our our bodies.

Most people don't drink sufficient water after which surprise why we go through crippling headaches, fatigue, weakness, loss of motivation and strength, sleep disturbances and simply can't get our mind straight. A tiny tweak is regularly all it takes.

Drink more water and see both your cognitive and physical performance shoot for the stars!

Get preserve of a reusable aluminum bottle and fill it with water, then sip from it frequently at some stage in the day. When it's empty fill it up once more and hold on sipping. You want to intention for no less than round 2-three liters in line with day for most suitable performance.

A super tip that a fitness enterprise colleague gave me turned into to offer myself small dreams at some stage in the day. In my case I intention to drink the contents of my 1 liter bottle earlier than midday each day after which drink at the least every other complete bottle withinside the afternoon. Add to this numerous cups of clean caffeine-unfastened natural tea, and there's no question that I'm hydrated, clear-minded and energized!

HABIT 9
Ditch Those Stimulants

You're suffering after a disturbed nights' sleep or mainly anxious day and you're determined for whatever that will help you live awake, increase your strength and assist you experience alert. So you attain for the answer which you recognize satisfactory - the double photographs of espresso, the again-to-again strength beverages and the limitless cups of strong, sugary, caffeinated tea.

And I'll come up with credit - it does paintings quite properly. Well, for a brief whilst at maximum.

But quickly after that caffeine load has hit your bloodstream, you begin to experience slower, much less centered and extra like a zombie once more. So, what do you do? You attain for extra caffeine, of course, and so the cycle continues.

When you eat those stimulants you're growing your tiers of pressure hormones (consisting of cortisol), which have an effect on your temper, your immune response, your heart, your blood strain and lots of different physical processes. You also can cause migraines, belly and digestive issues, and your blood sugar tiers will range wildly. As properly as all of this, stimulants are simply an synthetic manner of feeling suitable and aren't focused on the foundation of the problem.

This applies for all types of stimulants, consisting of espresso, tea, strength beverages, sugary sodas, cigarettes or prescription and non-prescription drugs. Stimulant dependency may be an pricey dependancy while you virtually reflect onconsideration on it.

So, why not try these healthier ways of feeling uplifted, energized and de-stressed instead?

• Gradually update your day by day espresso dependancy with inexperienced tea to lessen cravings and caffeine withdrawals (and ultimately update inexperienced tea together along with your favourite caffeine-unfastened tea alternative)

• Boost your consumption of clean end result and B-Vitamins to gasoline your frame of herbal strength

• Try the usage of carob to your warm beverages (as opposed to cocoa or cacao) as a
stimulant-unfastened chocolate alternative

• Go for a run or take a brisk stroll withinside the clean air

• Play your favourite upbeat and uplifting music

• Switch off all electronics and get an early night's sleep

• Go for a clean and healing swim. For satisfactory outcomes head for the sea!

HABIT 10
Power-Up On Carbs

As far as fashions go, the anti-carb movement must surely be one of the most damaging for your health, energy levels and happiness.

What different sort of food plan might have you ever keep away from one of the maximum critical foremost meals groups, and chance irreversibly detrimental you fitness, simply for vanity's sake?

Carbohydrates are without a doubt crucial for our bodily and intellectual fitness, and heading off them is reckless and unsafe. You see; carbohydrates are the number one supply of gas and electricity for the mind and frame. When we devour them, they get damaged down into glucose in our digestive systems. This glucose is a molecule that immediately feeds our mind tissues and our cells so we've the electricity to assume, move, thrive and survive. Glucose maintains us alive, simple and simple.

The hassle is that many so-referred to as fitness specialists have become their wholefood carbs careworn with the empty carbs. Not all carbs are created equally.

Choose unwisely and you may be loading your self up with exceptionally processed white bread, desserts and cookies that disrupt your blood sugar tiers and reason different similarly problems.

You want to get the ones wholesome carbs lower back for your existence with the aid of using deciding on wholegrain breads, brown rice, pasta, quinoa, candy potatoes, bananas, and beneficiant portions of sparkling fruit and veggies. *You mind and your soul will thanks for it!*

HABIT 11
Plan Your Meals

There isn't anyt any excuse to ever inn to exceptionally refined, additive and preservative weighted down meals that harm your fitness, pile at the extra pounds, make you experience horrible and drain you of electricity.

Even in case you slightly have time to breathe, there's a manner you may nevertheless make sure you're consuming a nutrient-dense weight loss plan so one can go away you feeling happy and nourished. Pre-getting ready your food, or specific elements, will assure you a wholesome, brief and fulfilling meal, even if matters get barely manic. The trick is withinside the making plans!

Why not pre-wash, chop or spiralize your vegetables in advance to save you time and energy after a busy day? You can also precook your roasted vegetables, rice and legumes to quickly bulk up a wholesome dish; or bag-up smoothie ingredients so they are ready to pull straight out of the freezer and into your blender. Also try creating your own trail mix by choosing your favorite nuts, seeds and dried fruits for a quick and easy snack.

Meal making plans doesn't imply your meals could be dull, uninspiring or bland - the selections are yours, and are endless. It will offer you with a plethora of wholesome, brief-to-use elements and a bendy define so that you don't arrive domestic to understand there's not anything fit for human consumption for your cupboards. By making plans ahead, you may be capable of save intelligently and continually have some thing nutritious and scrumptious to enjoy.

How To Plan Your Meals

Even the busiest of human beings can take ten mins or so as soon as every week to seize a chunk of paper and a pen and jot down the food and elements they would love to devour for the relaxation of the week. Simply write down the times of the week alongside one aspect and scribble your preferred food withinside the spot subsequent to every day, and you'll locate that meals purchasing turns into an entire lot easier. You simply want to shop for the elements for the food to your list, saving you crucial time and additionally money.

Don't assume you want to paste rigidly to those thoughts in case you extrade your thoughts midweek - virtually switch the times or test together along with your pre-organized elements to fit your tastes.

HABIT 12

Ditch Your Scales

The secret that no one wants to tell you about losing weight and regaining your happiness is simple. Ditch your scales, and vow never to weigh yourself again!

This may appear to be a loopy component to do. After all, how are you going to choose your development and maintain your self in test in case you don't have a device to degree with? The solution lies for your dating with meals.

When you weigh your self regularly, you're doing all the following matters:

• Placing your happiness, motivations and feel of manage on how a whole lot you weigh

• Judging and comparing your self esteem on that magical variety

• Focusing at the smaller, unimportant info while you want to be searching at the larger photograph alternatively

I can nearly listen you protest while you examine that list, however permit me to interrupt it down.

Your bodily weight doesn't be counted. What does be counted is the way you experience, how a whole lot dangerous frame fats you're carrying, the way you experience for your clothes, and what kind of electricity you've got got - now no longer a few arbitrary parent on a weighing device. You see, your weight varies wildly at special factors all through the day or maybe the month relying to your hydration, your muscle mass, how a whole lot you've got got eaten, whether or not you're ovulating, menstruating and so on. It isn't an correct mirrored image of your internal fitness or whether or not you want to lose weight.

When you examine the variety on a scale you robotically choose your self and how 'good' you've got got been that specific week; 'am I a achievement or a failure today?' Whilst your intentions are great, you're inadvertently trapping your self right into a cycle of yo-yo dieting, guilt and self-loathing, while alternatively you must be making wholesome way of life selections to help you regularly alter your weight to be able to maintain it off long-term.

So, study the larger picture. Ditch the scales and use how you're feeling as your manual in place of how lots you weigh. Do you sense cushty to your body? Are you healthy? How are your electricity degrees? All these items depend a ways extra than a number!

HABIT 13
Cook from Scratch

Get back to basics. Cook from scratch more often so you can gain 100% control over what you are putting into your body.

We simply don't realize the whole volume of the numerous nasties pumped into processed foods; from the fat and sugars to the additives, preservatives, GMO elements, environmentally destructive elements and chemicals. The most effective certain manner to keep away from all of that is to put together our meals ourselves.

Don't worry - you don't must be a gourmand chef or conjure up complex and time-ingesting recipes. Nor does it depend in case you slightly realize the way to fry an onion. All that topics is your preference to nourish your self with the very best exceptional vitamins and a willingness to examine new skills.

There are a few exquisite web sites accessible with the intention to educate you to make your favored food the usage of most effective herbal and healthful elements. Why now no longer appearance up a recipe to your favored meal and deliver it a try?

HABIT 14
Don't Forget Turmeric

Imagine if there has been simply one 'surprise remedy' you may use each unmarried day that might be cheap, convenient and now no longer require a go to for your pharmacist or fitness store. The first-class information you'll pay attention all day is that there may be one. *And its call is turmeric.*

Turmeric is the peppery spice that offers that acquainted vibrant yellow colour to curries and different spiced food. It additionally gives extra fitness blessings than you could imagine. Here are simply a number of them:

It's a effective anti inflammatory. Turmeric carries excessive degrees of a compound called curcumin, that's a effective anti inflammatory relatively powerful in treating situations which includes arthritis, Crohn's, ulcerative colitis and IBS with out inflicting nasty aspect effects.

It shrinks pre-cancerous lesions. The very equal compound, curcumin, has been discovered to reduce pre-cancerous lesions which includes polyps which could result in colon cancer.

It can assist beat Alzheimer's sickness. Curcumin additionally facilitates clean the mind of plaque accumulation, notion to be one of the main reasons of the sickness.

It facilitates combat cancer. Curcumin carries excessive degrees of antioxidants, which combat the loose radicals which could harm cells and purpose cancer. It also can assist save you any present cancers from spreading in addition for the duration of the body.

It improves your liver function. Turmeric facilitates to enhance the liver cleansing manner thru its antioxidant motion upon fats cells.

It improves coronary heart fitness. The curcumin that facilitates clean plaque from the mind additionally prevents plaque from gathering in the coronary heart and vascular system, as a consequence assisting lessen the danger of coronary heart sickness and stroke.

A little is going an extended manner, so sprinkle a sprint of this scrumptious surprise spice into your food to assist shield your self from sickness.

HABIT 15
Drink Hibiscus Tea

Hibiscus tea has recently been revealed to be somewhat of a natural 'wonder-drug', lowering blood pressure, easing hypertension, benefitting our brains, reducing inflammation and even tackling those free radicals which can lead to cancer and premature aging.

Hibiscus tea is powerfully wealthy in nutrition C and antioxidants, and higher still, tastes clearly fruity and scrumptious. So, in case you're seeking out an nearly effort-loose dependancy to assist rework your fitness and happiness, you higher get consuming!

Drinking caffeine-loose natural teas additionally offer a variety of different widespread blessings, which includes growing your consumption of water, lowering your intake of stimulants like tea and coffee, and additionally assisting to flush pollution out of your cells. For first-class results, you need to be consuming round to 3 cups of the stuff every day.

Before you sprint out and get a field of hibiscus tea, take a peep at any fruit or natural teas you may have mendacity round to your cupboards. Hibiscus seems in lots of blends so that you may already be taking part in its blessings with out realizing.

In fact, I suppose I'll make myself a brew proper now!

HABIT 16
Avoid Vitamin Deficiencies

Even with the healthiest of diets, all it takes is an oversight and a alternate in circumstances (or maybe of weather) and you could locate your self tormented by dietary deficiencies, that may purpose debilitating signs and ability long-time period harm. It's essential to have ordinary blood checks to make certain which you have all your bases included in case you need to save you this taking place to you.

The two most common vitamin deficiencies in the western world are vitamin B 12 and vitamin D.

Vitamin B 12

Vitamin B 12 is discovered nearly completely in merchandise of animal origin, However for the ones folks who lessen our animal meals intake for our average fitness, and for appropriate reason, it's far the only nutrition which could hard to get in case you devour a plant-wealthy diet. However, *anybody can grow to be nutrition* B 12 deficient, and it's now no longer some thing moderate which you have to ignore. Suffer from this and you may enjoy low power stages, terrible memory, confusion, tingling and numbness withinside the fingers and feet, and may subsequently reason lengthy-time period nerve harm and in excessive cases, even death. You can without difficulty cope with this danger via way of means of taking a diet B 12 complement in pill, liquid or injectable shape, plus frequently eating ingredients together with dietary yeast or B 12 fortified plant milks. Speak on your healthcare practitioner in case you require in addition advice.

Vitamin D

Thankfully, diet D is an entire lot less complicated to get and doesn't arise from dietary holes in our modern diets . You see diet D is to be had withinside the maximum fun shape of all - daylight. The movement of daylight on our pores and skin truly reasons our our bodies to provide greater diet D, maintaining us healthy, glad and strengthening our bones withinside the process.

However, many human beings live interior a ways an excessive amount of, slap on an excessive amount of sunscreen, and cowl up an excessive amount of in their pores and skin. Vitamin D deficiency can reason weakened bones, despair, weakness, weight gain, and if left untreated can reason a couple of sclerosis or cancer. Humans want daylight, simply as every other shape of lifestyles in this planet. So get accessible withinside the sparkling air and experience the solar to your pores and skin. If you stay in a cooler climate, paintings interior or discover your self to be diet D deficient, you could additionally take a plant-derived diet D complement in pill or liquid shape.

HABIT 17

Balance Your Hormones Naturally

A near pal of mine used to go through extraordinarily together along with her hormones. There wasn't a unmarried day that she didn't have a few associated fitness grievance or some other to deal with, from terrible cystic acne, to hair loss, to extra facial hair, to PMT, painful periods, weight gain, moderate despair and temper swings. She become tormented by polycystic ovary syndrome and not anything appeared to paintings. Her lifestyles become almost insufferable and after a few years of trying, she become slowly going for walks out of options.

That become till she grew to become to me.

I understood all too nicely the struggles she become going through, and collectively we evolved a sturdy and complete movement plan that converted her lifestyles completely. You can consider how glad she become.

If you're going through comparable struggles and are giving up hope, have confidence that there may be an answer accessible for you. It simply takes time.

The first actual issue you want to do is to test each your thyroid stages and hormone stages as these items can have an effect on each other and throw the whole lot else out of whack. Once you've got got diagnosed your problems, you may take steps to goal every in flip and subsequently start to experience better. Here are some crucial ones:

1. Limit your intake of omega-6's
2. Reduce your intake of caffeine
3. Avoid pollution and xenoestrogens
4. Get greater sleep
5. Take a complement together with Magnesium or Agnus Castus
6. Get everyday exercise

You can find more details on how to best implement remedies for your hormonal issues by reading my #1 seller: *Herbal Hormone Handbook.*

HABIT 18
Balance Work, Rest & Play

What do you suspect is the most important remorse that the death have approximately their lives? I'll come up with a clue; it is now no longer lacking their income goal in August 2015, neither is it lacking that advertising that they labored so difficult for, neither is it now no longer spending greater time on the office.

It's the remorse of now no longer grabbing lifestyles via way of means of the horns and residing in step with their very own goals and rules. It's the remorse of now no longer spending sufficient time with cherished ones, now no longer doing all the matters they definitely experience passionate approximately, and neglecting their very own needs. Imagine if that become you, mendacity there, with those varieties of regrets...

There is most effective one manner to keep away from struggling this fate, and this is to march on your very own drum.

Don't commit your whole lifestyles on your profession and finishing up neglecting positive factors of your lifestyles like your family, buddies or hobbies. Instead assume lengthy and difficult approximately what definitely topics to you, and if the lifestyles you're main doesn't suit up, you want to take movement.

Live up on your very own capability with regards to paintings, however additionally take entertainment withinside the easy pleasures in lifestyles. Revive your favored hobbies, or maybe take pleasure in all of these stuff you positioned withinside the 'someday' pile. Take time to disconnect from the world. Simply take a seat down again and take all of it in. We are most effective right here as soon as so your challenge can most effective be to stay and experience it.

How approximately your lifestyles proper now? Is it nicely balanced? Are your pouring an excessive amount of power into one place and neglecting others?

Be sincere with your self and make the adjustments you want to stay a higher brighter existence.

HABIT 19
Prioritize Pleasure

When was the last time you enjoyed yourself? *Really enjoyed yourself?* **The kind of enjoyment that makes you helplessly burst into laughter, makes your heart beat a little faster and makes your face muscles sore from all that smiling?**

It's so smooth to spend all our time ticking all of the boxes, looking after our careers and our households and our friends, but forgetting to take some time to attend to ourselves. Essentially, we have to be the maximum essential human beings in our lives and we want to prioritize our very own pride earlier than we even reflect onconsideration on giving to others. It's unexpected how this easy existence hack will raise your ranges of happiness and maintain them there.

Pleasure and the cappotential to revel in pride is one of the few matters that makes us uniquely human and we have to be indulging ourselves greater frequently to experience each happier and healthier.

So, have a few amusing and deal with your self. Dedicate at the least thirty mins every and each day to some thing you discover pleasurable, some thing that is probably and regardless of how small. For me, it's enjoyable on the give up of a protracted day with a splendid new ee-e book and a cup of natural tea.

What will convey you pride? What easy dependancy will you upload on your day to enhance your happiness potential?

HABIT 20
Develop a Morning Routine

Too a lot of us rush round from the very second we open our eyes. The alarm pulls us from our desires and we get stuck up in a whirlwind of rushed arrangements for the day, chaos and confusion and stress, and spend some distance an excessive amount of time searching the auto keys, deciding on what to wear, wrestling the children into suitable apparel or asking them to sweep their teeth. It's making me experience frazzled simply considering it!

Now consider you can begin your day in an entire unique manner. Imagine you can wake slowly, welcome the morning with open fingers and lightly blow the cobwebs of sleep farfar from your body. Imagine a calm, soothing, non violent begin to the day. Sounds awesome, doesn't it?

You could make this dream turn out to be a fact via way of means of converting the manner you examine your morning and beginning a few new wholesome behavior so that it will take your temper from careworn to soothed.

Here's what you need to do:

• Collect and put together the whole lot that you'll want on your day the night time earlier than

• Wake at the least ten mins in advance and provide your self greater time to clean your thoughts and accumulate your mind earlier than you release out of bed

• Use this time to mirror and ask your self what you're thankful for, to inspire a nice mindset (see 'Habit 26' for greater detail)

• Start the day proper via way of means of making the time to experience a quick yoga session, a chain of stretches, nice affirmations or meditation

• Mentally plan out your day at the same time as you're withinside the bathe and uninterrupted - consciousness for your priorities first

• Make time to experience a wholesome and healthful breakfast, inclusive of oatmeal with sparkling berries, to gas you for the day ahead

Implementing a 'slow' morning recurring instead of a tensed, careworn one will assist you and your own circle of relatives begin the day with a grin and an air of positivity.

HABIT 21
Yield in Your Favorite Music

Music touches our souls. It makes us feel good, it evokes long-forgotten memories and emotions and it lifts our spirits like nothing else.

Remember that antique music you used to adore? You recognize the one. As quickly because the acquainted riff met your eardrums, a grin could unfold throughout your face. You should in no way flip that music off till it reached the very give up, or even then the temptation to re-concentrate became difficult to resist!

And absolute confidence you've as soon as had a tune that could raise your power and motivation, and go away you feeling pumped and equipped to stand something that existence could throw at you. Or a tune that might lessen you to tears inside only some bars? Or a tune that might assist you neglect about approximately your problems for simply one second, and raise you to brighter, happier places?

But you likely don't concentrate to it anymore. Your existence may also have turn out to be too demanding and you've got different commitments and jobs to attend to now. But here's the thing - in case you need to inject a few immediate pride again into your existence, elevate your spirits and raise your stage of wellbeing, you want to restore that track series and experience the ones nostalgic sounds.

Music has the strength to at once have an effect on our brains and tweak our emotions, which we will harness to advantage our very own day by day lives. Simply increase the dependancy of being attentive to greater track as you move approximately your day. This would possibly suggest being attentive to a splendid playlist as you dress withinside the morning, or while you commute, or while you consume lunch, prepare dinner dinner or maybe loosen up withinside the evening.
Whatever works for you, works on your soul too.

So why now no longer rediscover your antique favorites, find out a few splendid new sounds and praise your self with an uplifting day?

Tell me, what track haven't you listened to in a at the same time as?

HABIT 22
Find Your Tribe

Humans are social creatures. Without positive, social touch and guide we absolutely wither and lose ourselves. You simplest want to don't forget the plight of the aged who regularly locate themselves housebound and with out traffic for days, if now no longer weeks, on quit. Just consider what type of impact this has upon them.

If we don't have supportive people around us, we feel detached, misunderstood and lonely.

But if you have your personal tribe of buddies round to guide you, lifestyles will in no way be the equal again. They will come up with the energy to realise your wildest desires and face up to the worst matters that lifestyles can throw at you. You will sense cherished and understood for the specific man or woman which you are, regardless of what you've got got or what you do. It's approximately locating human beings that percentage your view of the sector and might effortlessly recognize your angle of the sector.

Finding Friends As Adults

Once we depart excessive college or university and develop older, it is able to be a lot tougher to locate folks that ought to shape those tribes. *Don't worry - we have got all been there.* But wherein are we able to locate them? What must we are saying to them whilst we do locate them? And how can we create significant relationships with the ones round us?

In real fact, locating buddies as an person is lots like dating. You want to get your self obtainable and be open to the sector and what it has to provide with out being overly concerned approximately the final results, regardless of how critical that final results would possibly sense to you proper now. You might also additionally sense a touch shy or dubious on the start, however consider that everyone feels this manner.

Talk to human beings anywhere you go, although that's simply to the neighborhood library. You'll be amazed at who you may meet in there. And via way of means of complimenting someone's hair or shoes, you could simply brighten their day.

Don't cut price the concept of becoming a member of a class, taking on a brand new interest or maybe reviving an antique one. By doing this you could meet like-minded human beings with comparable interests, providing you with the precise conversational subject matter to assist 'smash the ice'. You'll construct your personal happiness in addition to locating your tribe. Just attempt it out.

What one factor ought to you do to fulfill greater like-minded human beings? Take a while to contemplate this query after which take action!

HABIT 23
Feed Your Mind

Ever because the second you had been born, your interest and thirst for know-how has been packing your mind complete of useful (and now no longer-so-useful) portions of statistics. You've been studying and developing for so long as you may consider and it maintains you sharp and intelligent.

However, withinside the current age of statistics saturation, we regularly search for a brief restoration in social media or fact tv shows. You would possibly revel in these items and locate they assist you to loosen up and disconnect on the quit of an extended difficult day, and this is great, on occasion. But doing this too regularly is losing a while and permitting the rot to set in. Don't allow your mind flip stagnant and permit boredom and restlessness to seep in.

If you permit your self to often devour this 'chewing gum for the mind' then you'll observe that your cognitive capacity diminishes, your private know-how and increase involves a entire standstill and you may in no way pretty make your desires come true. Your lifestyles must be a adventure toward self-achievement and the simplest manner you may do that is to maintain studying and developing.

So in place of losing hour upon hour in the front of the TV, dropping hours in the front of Facebook or YouTube and spending time gossiping approximately the lives of the wealthy and famous, awareness in your private improvement instead.

Grab a brilliant book on a subject that fascinates you, vow to finally learn that second language, enroll in a course at your local college, learn to dance salsa, paint a picture, visit new places, or begin a great meditation habit and watch yourself bloom. Read as much as possible,

exercise whole-hearted curiosity in the world, ask questions and seek answers, and think deeply about the things that matter most to you.

Reading especially facilitates stimulates the mind, improves your reminiscence and awareness, reduces pressure and expands your vocabulary. The greater talents and know-how you obtain, the higher you may address the various demanding situations that lifestyles might also additionally throw at you.

HABIT 24
Build Self-Love & Positivity

Many of us don't love ourselves quite enough.

We declare we're doing fine, we paintings toward being kinder and greater forgiving of ourselves and of our actions. But can we truely love ourselves?

It appears altogether too narcissistic to sense 'self-love' and it's type of embarrassing too. We ward off the subject, wondering that we're now no longer deserving sufficient of our personal love, or wondering that we're simplest authorized to like the ones round us and now no longer ourselves.

But that is a part of the trouble we've with our happiness and experience of achievement. Inject a touch self-love and positivity into your lifestyles via way of means of fostering a few healthful habits, and you may reap a lot greater than you've got ever imagined.

Don't accept as true with me? Then allow's consider what takes place whilst you don't love your self.

When You Don't Love Yourself Enough

Consider that internal voice that silently passes touch upon your conduct and your attitude, for ever and ever trying to sabotage your achievement and your happiness. It drums it into your head which you are come what may substandard, unlovable, a failure, a fraud and every other bad adjective you may suppose of. It tells you that your worst-case situation will possibly come real and could make a mountain out of a molehill. Now what type of lifestyles is this? Living as a sufferer of that internal voice that has no foundation in reality by any means and best serves to carry you down.

You would possibly suppose that there may be no get away from this terrible voice and that it's simply the way you have been made, however I actually have to inform you proper now which you are wrong. Utterly wrong.

The distinction among the effective folks who love themselves and the bad who dislike their personal life comes right all the way down to best one thing; how carefully they concentrate to that internal voice of negativity.

The effective ones recognise the reality and brush away the lies this voice would possibly whisper, and the bad ones avidly concentrate to each phrase and take them as law, restricting themselves and their conduct withinside the process.

How To Find Your Self-Love

I don't need you to be this type of folks who in no way obtain their desires because of the iron-like grip of this voice. Nothing on your lifestyles will ever enhance in case you retain to allow it dominate your lifestyles.

The adventure closer to fostering self-love and positivity is simpler stated than done, however with the subsequent few tips, you'll be amazed simply how without problems it comes.

1) Every day inform your self you're notable and worth of all that the arena has to offer. Look into the mirror, gaze into your eyes and remind your self how notable you clearly are.

2) Take a while to mirror in your lifestyles and the arena round you. Through mirrored image we will discover ways to discover our bad behavior and broaden greater effective ones.

3) Don't evaluate your self to others. You are unique. You are beautiful. There isn't anyt any one such as you withinside the world, and this is amazing.

4) Develop a thicker pores and skin and don't take the movements of others too personally. It's possibly now no longer approximately you at all, however as an alternative their temper or their personal private instances which you're now no longer conscious of.

5) Banish that sufferer mentality. You are chargeable for your movements, nobody else. Nor are you accountable for the movements of others.

Practice those steps and you'll be astonished at how lots higher you experience and simply how quick you may educate your mind into loving your self increasingly every day.

HABIT 25
Strive for Your Goals

Without a map, how do any of us know where we're going? How can we really make our wildest dreams and perfect life become a technicolor reality? How can we meet the challenges that life might throw our way if we are blind to the future?

Of path we will't. Yet lots of us stay our lives on this shortsighted manner. We amble on aimlessly, hoping that some thing thrilling and amusing can be simply across the nook with out ever status up and grabbing lifestyles with the aid of using the horns. Success and happiness doesn't simply fall into all people's lap - you've were given to make it happen. And meaning placing your self a few thrilling dreams.

Goal-placing will assist you destroy loose from the monotony of lifestyles, declare the lifestyles you need to steer and hold you urgent onwards and upwards whilst matters get tough.

Defining Your Goals

What subjects to you may glaringly vary from that of your great friend, your accomplice or your parents, so it's as much as you to determine precisely what those dreams can be. So take a while and do not forget what clearly subjects to you.

Where do you see yourself in a year's time? How about five years? Or even ten? Where do you want to be? And who with?

Set your self short-time period and long-time period dreams after which clearly make it happen. If you're having problem with doing this exercise, why now no longer suppose as an alternative approximately what you will hate to be doing? What might be your worst nightmare?
This is the trick that shifts me from uncertain to targeted and driven.

Making Them Happen

Once you've got got mentioned your dreams, destroy them down into smaller short-time period objectives and do not forget how you may flow closer to

them. Keep your self

accountable. Think approximately them often, communicate approximately them to all people who will concentrate and fill your each waking second with desires of all of it turning into real. You may want to even extrade your computer wallpaper to an inspiring photo associated with certainly considered one among your dreams or maybe create a imaginative and prescient board.

Dream massive and your lifestyles turns into simply as massive!

HABIT 26
Count Your Blessings

When you awaken withinside the morning, what's the primary idea that passes thru your brain? Is it certainly considered one among marvel that that is the begin of any other day, or do you drag your self off the bed in dread for what lies ahead? You desire you didn't have your stupid task together along with your stupid colleagues, you desire you have been taller or extra appealing or didn't want to put on spectacles. You simply desire the entirety was… well, specific by some means.

These very mind are exactly what are status among you and a great existence, and also you want to increase a gratitude exercise in case you are ever to sense happy.

You see, it's all approximately perspective.

Perspective

Ask your self proper now, what's the distinction among the wealthy westerner who has all of it however is by some means depressed and the poverty-troubled catastrophe survivor who has misplaced all of it however nonetheless smiles? Perspective.

If you have a take a observe the entirety you haven't were given and rely the methods your existence is horrible and remind your self which you are so extraordinarily sad, your existence might be much like that. You will sense deprived, horrible and sad due to the fact you're specializing in what you understand your self to be lacking.

But if rather you make the effort to comprehend the stuff you do have, the methods that the sector has blessed you and sense grateful for the entirety you've were given, you may clearly sense appreciative, blessed and grateful. It's like swapping a lens.

Look for the poor and you'll see poor. Look for the fantastic and you may be beaten with the splendor of your existence.

Because even in case you sense at this second which you don't have anything to be grateful for, I promise you which you do, irrespective of how small it'd be. And the

extra you search for your advantages, the extra you may find out and you'll sense in reality thankful.

Becoming More Grateful

To get started, actually rely the ones advantages of yours. At the start or cease of every day, take a few paper and write down as a minimum three matters that you are feeling thankful for. These can be the equal matters each day, such as "I sense blessed that I even have the possibility to do paintings I love" or "I sense blessed to have a lovely family". Repetition is okay - the strength of this workout lies to your very own idea procedure and now no longer the completed result. Then repeat this for as a minimum 30 days (or maybe longer) and you'll note the fantastic distinction to your existence.

HABIT 27
Get Moving

It's the cease of any other day and I'm feeling guilty. I realize I've spent a long way an excessive amount of time placing the completing touches to this ee-e book and meaning that as plenty as I've had a tremendous day, I've additionally been sitting proper right here in the front of my pc display and feature slightly moved a muscle.

I realize that if I spend the relaxation of my day like this, I will turn out to be feeling slow and lethargic, heavy and demotivated and I may have lousy hassle falling asleep. Continue for plenty longer and I should get depressed, fall prey to all the viruses doing the rounds, pile on lots of extra weight and commonly sense horrible.

That's due to the fact our our bodies have been constructed to move, and if we don't get the workout that our our bodies want, our fitness will go through immensely. I don't plan on letting that show up whenever soon.

Once my operating day is done, I won't simply flop in the front of the television. I need to get available into the sparkling air and get transferring so I can enhance my circulation, guard my fitness and sense top notch and energized as soon as again. But that doesn't imply that I'll sweat it out with all the different fitness center bunnies. I'm now no longer that form of girl. I can nonetheless revel in the advantages of workout via way of means of doing the matters that I love, and you could too.

So, what activities do you like doing? Is there a sport that you adore? A sport you used to adore but haven't found time for lately? I'd urge you to get out there and do it. All it takes is just 30 minutes per day.

Personally I'm keen on walking, cycling, dancing and swimming as they're masses of a laugh and slightly sense like workout at all. What might do it for you?

HABIT 28
Sleep Yourself Stronger

'Life is simply too brief to spend it napping.' Isn't that how the announcing goes? But I'd beg to differ.

In fact, I'd clearly say that existence is simply too brief to spend sleep-deprived, running at much less than your complete potential, lethargic, indifferent and lacking out on a life-time of adventures due to the fact you're too tired. Who wishes loopy subtle sugar cravings and contamination without a doubt due to the fact you aren't napping enough?

I recognize that there are too many distractions and too many stuff to do. We all lead busy lives with slightly any time to say again and so it's comprehensible that we live up too past due in an try and trap up with ourselves.

But that is skewed logic. We may want to paintings a long way extra efficiently, attaining extra, knocking off extra duties from our 'to do lists' and now have beneficiant quantities of time left for a laugh on the quit if we best get our sleep.

Sleep is the ultimate anti-aging solution that energizes our bodies, boosts our brains, heals chronic health conditions, helps regulate our

metabolism, reduces cravings and even helps you lose weight in the process. What's not to like about it?

Starting from proper now, make a promise to your self that you'll begin getting the sleep your thoughts and frame deserves. For maximum human beings that is round 8 hours, however you may locate that barely extra or maybe barely much less works higher for you. You will sincerely note the difference!

HABIT 29
Master Minimalism

For a few unusual reason, a whole lot of the sector considers a person's possessions to be the first-rate signal of success. The larger your own home, the quicker your car, the extra rooms you want to shop you junk the higher, proper? Well simply, no.

Most of these things is bought as a deal with however finally ends up as an absolute burden after a while. We spend precious entertainment time organizing our stuff, cleansing our stuff, retaining our stuff or even running more difficult and having much less of a actual lifestyles on the way to earn extra cash to get extra of these things. It's using us loopy and it really has to stop.

The time has come to dispose of your 'stuff'.

You understand, that stuff that clutters your closet and dominates you time. You can be loose from all of it and notice your pleasant of lifestyles undergo the roof.

Because stuff doesn't really matter, even if the clever ad campaigns tell us it does. What matters is our happiness, our health, our relationships, our enjoyment of life and the degree to which we can achieve our wildest dreams.

You understand I'm talking experience here.

Stuff is simply stuff. It provides no cost, reasons strain and we will't take it with us while we die, notwithstanding what the historic Egyptians may have thought.

Become A Minimalist

So have the first-rate spring-easy of your whole lifestyles. Sell or donate undesirable possessions, get rid of clutter, reorganize your area and best hold the matters that actually upload cost in your lifestyles. *A clean area = a clean thoughts!*

A extraordinary manner to get began out is to goal to donate or promote at the least one undesirable ownership each day. Perhaps hold a container for goodwill withinside the nook of your hallway and each day pop some thing inside. There can be a person someplace that definitely wishes what you need to offer, so move beforehand and

provide lower back to the sector.

Another right method you could strive is to address one precise region of your own home and easy it out completely. You may determine to begin with the lowest drawer to your bedroom, so that you undergo each unmarried object and determine whether or not it truely provides cost in your lifestyles. If it does, fine, pop it lower back inside. If it doesn't then it's time to promote or donate it.

Over the years, I've slowly decreased my possessions to a possible stage and I can hopefully say that my pleasant of lifestyles has in no way been higher. Why don't you provide it a move?

HABIT 30
Tackle Stress

Stress is a killer.

It poses critical stress upon your intellectual and bodily fitness and ruins your lifestyles. Who desires to stay in moved quickly and frantic manner? I understand I genuinely don't. Stress feels horrible and does horrible matters to you, so in case you need to stay a top notch lifestyles, you want to broaden wholesome behavior on the subject of managing strain.

Stress can make a contribution to depression, coronary heart attacks, excessive blood pressure, consolation eating, weight-advantage toothaches, migraines, speech problems, slumbering problems, forgetfulness, anxiety, irritated outbursts, panic attacks, lies, nightmares, and extra.

It additionally locations a massive burden at the adrenal glands, which could throw your hormones out of balance, reason you to maintain directly to weight, make your hair fall out and irritate an entire host of different signs and symptoms which include asthma, eczema and psoriasis.

And it a long time you past your years, can reason you to consolation eat, mistreat your family and sooner or later hit burnout.

But What Can We Do About It?

But it's now no longer as though we will begin dwelling in a defensive bubble loose from all varieties of strain. In fact, small quantities of strain are taken into consideration to be superb and motivating. But it's while it receives out of manipulate and the way we address it that counts.

For an extended time, I determined it truely difficult to procedure my strain in superb ways, and once in a while my efforts could simply make matters worse for me, and now no longer higher. But I quickly observed quite a number wholesome behavior that helped me to get the whole lot below manipulate and now have a heap of a laugh.

Why don't you strive the subsequent behavior to address your strain?

Try meditation. Meditation lets in you disconnect from the sector and discover a diploma of internal calm. It works wonders on strain and additionally depression, and isn't simply for 'hippies' because it become as soon as perceived. Give it a strive.

Practice yoga. Yoga is a shape of shifting meditation. It improves your mind-frame connection and stretches out your muscle tissues which could keep large quantities of strain and tension. It may even assist you sleep like a baby!

Start journaling. Get your mind out and onto a web page with out worry of being judged through the ones round you. Just begin writing!

Take up running. Running is a extraordinary manner to de-strain because it offers an outlet for all the strain hormones that gather inside our our bodies, that could doubtlessly reason bad fitness. Plus even as you run, you furthermore mght get out into the sparkling air and feature lots of time to suppose and reflect.

Enjoy a brand new innovative hobby. There's not anything pretty as healing as getting innovative. So, begin a writing exercise again, take in painting, drawing or sculpting, or maybe dig out that musical tool and lose your self in music.

CHAPTER 1
What is the Alkaline Diet?

The alkaline weight loss plan is absolutely one of a kind from all of these fad diets and poorly devised consuming plans that entice human beings right into a fake feel of hope. It's now no longer a idea this is primarily based totally on pseudo-technological know-how or present day consuming trends, however rather is primarily based totally on proof and good, difficult technological know-how. Each and all of us who trips toward accomplishing their frame's premiere pH stability (and doesn't stop alongside the manner!) can obtain wonderful blessings. You might be one of these human beings. You may want to revamp your fitness, reclaim your vitality, appearance definitely wonderful and rid your self of these fitness situations which can be so difficult to shift. You recognise those I mean - the pores and skin situations that withstand treatment, the IBS signs that continuously flare up, the allergies, the fatigue and the clouded thinking.
You CAN take away all of this through following the alkaline weight loss plan.

Studies finished through the Preventive Medicine Research Institute in Sausalito, California determined that most cancers sufferers following an alkalizing plant-primarily based totally weight loss plan misplaced weight, decreased their blood pressure, and healed an entire host of continual fitness issues further to really turning off numerous of the genes worried withinside the improvement of cancers. We simply can't forget about the terrific long-time period blessings that this life-style has to offer.

So, what precisely is the alkaline weight loss plan? What does it involve? And how can it enhance your fitness, beginning proper right here and now? Let's take a appearance.

What is Alkalinity?

First off, permit me give an explanation for the idea of alkalinity to you, with out dull you through delving too deeply into the clinical stuff.

You're likely acquainted with the concept of alkalinity and acidity out of your excessive faculty technological know-how class, and it's miles that very equal concept that we're coping with right here. Liquids may be measured in step with their alkalinity and acidity, and to this, we use a scale referred to as

a pH price that levels from 0-14. 0-7 is
acidic and more than 7 is alkaline.

Every residing issue wishes to have the precise pH stability so that it will stay healthily and feature best; fish require water with the precise pH ranges to survive, even as vegetation will thrive and flourish in pH balanced soil. Of course, this actual belief applies to our our bodies too. Our frame's blood, fluids and tissues require a pH price of about 7.365 so that it will feature at premier ranges - that is barely at the alkaline aspect of the scale. When the frame reaches this ideal acidity-alkalinity stability, it's miles much less liable to decreased immunity, continual ailment and cell damage.

pH Levels of the Blood

Death	Acidosis	Normal pH	Alkalosis	Death
6	7	7.34	7.38	7.8	9

Our our bodies have evolved to continuously shift and alter to hold homeostasis (stability) in all components of the frame, and it does the very equal issue for our pH ranges. Under herbal situations, it does a quite wonderful process at it too.

But the trouble is, the majority of us aren't living under these 'natural conditions'.

In our cutting-edge society, we eat 'foods' that our ancestors could slightly have recognized - the rather processed, saturated fats primarily based totally, refined-sugar food that make us slowly get sicker and sicker. And we issue our our bodies to a load of poisonous environmental factors: unnatural ranges of strain, abusing ourselves with stimulants, alcohol and drugs, poisoning ourselves with pesticides, pollutants and chemicals, and depriving ourselves of sleep; but we surprise why don't experience or appearance our best.

When we exercise those behaviors, we growth the acidity ranges in our systems, overloading the cleansing and alkalizing capabilities of the frame and developing a burden of irritation and sickness - together with acne, *pores and skin diseases, bowel issues, tumors, migraines, sound asleep troubles, mind fog, extra weight, infertility, depression*, and down the road, possibly some thing greater severe like coronary heart ailment or most cancers.

According to the American Journal of Clinical Nutrition, the fitness issues related to food regimen 'constitute through a long way the maximum extreme risk to public fitness'. They upload that 65% of adults over the age of 20 are obese, and 33% of all most cancers diagnoses are the end result of terrible food regimen and nutrition, together with obesity.

Sadly, our current diets and existence are slowly killing us and we want to do something positive about it earlier than it's too late.

What is the Alkaline Diet?

Enter the alkaline food regimen: the answer to attaining that ideal pH stability and reclaiming higher fitness and happiness.

Enthusiasts of the alkaline diet boast its benefits for:

• Youthful, clean skin (discount in getting older and removal of acne)

• Improved digestion and much less bloating

• Abundant power and faded fatigue

• Sustainable, long-time period weight loss

• More restful sleep

• Improved immunity (fewer colds and infections)

• Reduction in aches and pains (along with arthritis, gout and headaches)

• Increased intellectual readability and alertness

• Improvement in temper and happiness level

• Decreased danger of growing osteoporosis (acidity reasons minerals to be leeched from the bones to assist alkalise the blood)

• Reduction in danger of growing most cancers (alkalinity promotes healthful cell metabolism which is fundamental in most cancers prevention)

• Prevention and reversal of a number of continual diseases

The alkaline food regimen (and lifestyle) is set fending off toxic, acidifying ingredients and changing them with scrumptious, colourful ingredients that improve your nutrition, assist you shed extra weight and maximum importantly, rebalance your pH to achieve and
keep precise fitness.

When you eat, your meals is digested then damaged down through the kidneys into an alkaline or acidic base. This has a large effect upon the pH stability for your frame, and could create extra acidic or alkaline conditions, relying on what you're eating. Keep in thoughts that structurally 'acidic' ingredients don't always create an acidic environment (apple cider vinegar, *for example, has an alkalizing impact upon the frame) - it relies upon how the meals interacts with the frame as soon as metabolized.*

The alkaline idea entails ditching processed, delicate-sugar and excessive-fat 'empty' ingredients and changing them with an abundance of sparkling ingredients, simply as nature intended. You have nearly unfastened reign over a number of scrumptious sparkling culmination and greens (other than a few), lots of inexperienced leafy greens and seaweeds, sure nuts and seeds, healthful fats, healthful grains, spices and herbs. (Turn to the FREE BONUS recipe phase on the quit of this ee-e book to find out which scrumptious smoothies, *juices, teas, tonics and drinks you may revel in that encompass those outstanding ingredients.)*

The concept is to lessen acidic ingredients that purpose the frame to 'paintings in overdrive' to manner mistaken fuel. These encompass ingredients encompass wheat and gluten, animal-derived ingredients, caffeine, delicate sugar, alcohol and processed ingredients. But don't worry - this doesn't imply you want to cast off sure ingredients forever. You may be bendy for your method to the restoration ingredients you're setting into your frame, and intention for a stability of round 80/20 alkaline- acidic ingredients to your plate. That way, you may take pleasure in a few more healthy acid-forming ingredients (plant reassets are best, along with the occasional serving of oats, rice or cashews) with out feeling responsible or equipped to quit.

And it's now no longer simply your food regimen that desires a revamp in case you are tormented by excessive stages of acidity. Lifestyle conduct along with smoking, drinking, taking drugs, now no longer getting sufficient sleep or exercise, tormented by excessive stages of stress, and taking medicinal drugs can all create acidity withinside the frame. In addition to all of this, there also are numerous herbs, spices and dietary supplements that you may use to sell alkalinity and assist you for the duration of your restoration manner, which we are able to cope with in element for the duration of this ee-e book.

The concept that acidity reasons illness is a long way from being a brand new concept. In fact, acidosis (an excessively acidic frame) is a extensively studied phenomenon, and has extra these days been researched through Dr. Joseph Pizzorno. In his article posted withinside the British Journal of Nutrition (2009), he gives proof that a terrible food regimen reasons acidosis, and as a end result, results in an array of ailments and disease.

So, why is alkalinity so critical for first rate fitness? And what occurs while excessive acidity stages start to have an effect on your best of life? Let's delve into this withinside the following chapter.

CHAPTER 2
Alkalinity and Health

Now which you understand the basics of the alkaline weight loss program and life-style, it's time to dig a touch deeper into knowledge precisely why alkalinity is so critical for max fitness. We may also look at what sort of harm happens in the frame while your pH stability is disrupted, and why acidity is the basis purpose of the persistent disorder this is epidemic at some stage in the world.
Are you too acidic?

Why Alkalinity Matters

As we've got simply discovered, alkalinity subjects. It subjects due to the fact your frame desires to be barely alkaline to preserve ultimate fitness, heal and thrive - while an excessive amount of acidity acts because the breeding floor for negative fitness, disorder, and a slew of sick symptoms.

If you've got got an acidic frame, your digestion and GI fitness suffers, hindering the absorption of critical vitamins, minerals and phytonutrients to nourish and feed your tissues. Oxygen ranges withinside the blood drop, leaving you feeling fatigued and acting underneath par, and blood sugar ranges can vary wildly. All of this encourages your frame to save fats - and to pinnacle this off, extra acid is saved in the fats cells (making it more difficult as a way to lose weight). It's a vicious cycle!

The Damage that Acidity Inflicts

Acidosis doesn't simply make it extra tough on your frame to function; it clearly reasons incredible ranges of deterioration and harm, which luckily, may be reversed in case you trap it early enough. Here are simply a number of the bad influences of acidity:

Leeching minerals from the bones

In its try and rebalance excessive ranges of acidity, your frame turns to 2 minerals: calcium and magnesium. It borrows them from different components of your frame, stealing them from locations like your bones and brain, and leaving them weakened and extra susceptible to osteoporosis.

Free-radical damage

Acidic situations lessen the impact of antioxidants and growth the impact of dangerous unfastened radicals which could harm DNA, mobileular shape and reproduction, main to cancers, dementia, Alzheimer's disorder and plenty extra.

Accelerated aging

You'll appearance older that your years when you have a tremendously acidic frame. This is because of mobileular wall harm and the dearth of vitamins and oxygen that your pores and skin desires to repair, rejuvenate and live searching younger and fresh.

Fatigue

If you're too acidic, your frame works in overdrive to preserve the proper pH stability to sell oxygen waft and nutrient absorption, therefore leaving our our bodies in an exhausted, weakened state.

Growth of bacteria, fungi, molds, yeasts (including candida) and viruses

Highly acidic environments are the proper breeding floor for a large number of bacteria, fungi, molds, yeasts and viruses, all of which scouse borrow the vitamins out of your frame and are accountable for an entire host of fitness situations.

Health Problems that Acidity Creates

Here are simply a number of the fitness problems which can be associated with a pH imbalance withinside the frame:

- Heart disease or cardiovascular damage
-

High blood pressure

- Angina
- Obesity and weight gain

- Diabetes

- Bladder infections

- Kidney infections

- Kidney stones

- Lowered immunity

- Low energy

- Chronic fatigue syndrome

- Fibromyalgia

- Acne

- Osteoporosis

- Bone spurs

- Bone fractures

- Insomnia

- Allergies

- Eczema

- Psoriasis

- Hair loss

- Hormonal problems

- PMT

- Polycystic ovary syndrome
- Joint or muscular pain

Arthritis

- Gout

- Cancer

- Migraines and headaches

- Easily stressed or anxious

- Depression, lack of drive

- Digestive issues

- Gluten intolerance

- Insulin resistance

These are only a handful of the situations that an imbalance to your pH ranges can purpose. Acidity kills, and it's as much as you to convert your life. Only you could get to the lowest of the problem and assist your self to heal from the interior out.

In the following bankruptcy we can positioned the whole lot we've found out thus far into exercise and transfer the point of interest onto ourselves. How do our very own pH ranges suit up? What are the symptoms and symptoms of an acidic frame, and what are the reasons? Let's locate out.

CHAPTER 3
Your Body and Acidity

We now understand that the proper pH ranges of the human frame is about 7.365, and we understand that we want to take important steps to preserve this stability to make certain we revel in ideal fitness and wellbeing. But till now, it's all been as a substitute impersonal and theoretical. It's time to alternate all of that. After all, you're maximum inquisitive about how this all suits into your specific life-style and the way you could positioned all of it into exercise to revel in the advantages of this first-rate life-style.

Before you start your transformative journey, it's critical that we apprehend how we were given to have an acidic frame withinside the first place. Let's examine what reasons an acidic frame, the telltale symptoms and symptoms of an acidic frame, and the way to check our pH ranges. Are your fitness problems a end result of acidity?

What Causes an Acidic Body?

It's pretty regular for our our bodies to create many types of acids over the path of the day, like while we breathe, while we eat, while we exercise, while we speak and while we really simply 'live' - and additionally the ones produced from different kinds of metabolic processes. These don't purpose any types of troubles on your frame, because it really neutralizes them earlier than wearing on with different functions.

However, in case you are dwelling an bad lifestyle, ingesting acid-forming ingredients or maybe laid low with a critical fitness circumstance which includes most cancers or kidney failure, those tiers can quickly increase to unforgiving tiers, giving upward push to some thing from minor fitness issues to life-threatening acidosis.

We glaringly need to keep away from this from going on and want to take steps to dispose of triggers earlier than we start our direction toward healing. So what reasons your frame to grow to be acidic, and why? Let's take a look.

Your Eating Habits

There are many stuff that may reason an acidic frame and result in degenerative
diseases - and with out a shadow of a doubt, food regimen is the worst culprit, in particular the present day SAD or fashionable American food regimen that many humans exist on. These distinctly processed and excessive saturated fats ingredients aren't simply horrific to your waistline, your mood, your pores and skin and your strength tiers, they also can create a distinctly acidic surroundings wherein disease, bacteria, fungus and viruses can flourish.

But as noted earlier, food regimen isn't the handiest culprit withinside the list. After all, you may devour all of the proper form of ingredients however in case you're now no longer treating your frame holistically and paying attention to your lifestyle, you'll nonetheless face demanding situations in reversing the outcomes of acidity.

Other elements that make contributions to an acidic frame include:

Not enough sleep

When you burn the candle at each ends, your frame misses a important possibility to repair, rejuvenate and additionally manner pollution that it has encountered over the route of the day. If you're now no longer getting sufficient hours in, you're now no longer giving your frame the assist it desires to rebalance and obtain alkaline reputation again.

Drinking alcohol

Alcohol poses issues to our our bodies. Firstly, alcohol is a toxin that locations stress at the frame's organs, which includes the liver and the kidneys, so one can restrict the herbal pH neutralization manner and result in poisonous build-up of acidity. Secondly, alcohol simply will increase the manufacturing of belly acid inflicting each inner issues which includes ulcers, and of route a excessive acidity stage in the complete frame.

High levels of stress

Stress is a killer. When you're stressed, your frame will launch excessive tiers of the pressure hormones cortisol and noradrenaline for you to address the perceived threat. In historic instances those hormones could have helped us to bodily get away danger, while it now has a tendency to be mental and emotional elements that area pressure upon our our bodies. This may not appear to make plenty of a distinction from the outside, however from the inner, it's a very exclusive matter. These hormones won't have the risk to be expelled thru bodily motion and so that they stay inner our our bodies, collect in our tissues and lift our typical acid load, taking our pH to risky tiers.

After a brief length of time, pressure simply turns into a vicious cycle of acidity. Initial tiers of acidity reason irritation, and this irritation reasons illness, ache and suffering. This in flip reasons extra pressure, which will increase the tiers of acidity withinside the frame and reasons even extra irritation.

Food intolerances

A meals intolerance is your frame's sign this is isn't satisfied approximately some thing you've eaten, and it assaults the meals similar to it might a overseas invader with the acquainted signs of bloating, hives, a runny nose, sneezing, diarrhea, IBS, asthma, migraines and extra. When your frame reacts on this way, it's miles setting extra stress in your immune gadget and growing the acidity tiers for your frame as a result.

Over or under exercising

It's clearly critical to get the proper quantity of workout. Too little reasons our our bodies to slide into bad fitness, slows down our physical functions, reasons us to benefit weight, go through with bad stream and additionally prevents the frame from processing regular tiers of acidity and regaining stability effectively.

But don't throw your self into doing immoderate quantities of workout either - an excessive amount of may be simply as damaging. Any form of bodily workout increases tiers of lactic acid, that's the reason of these sore muscle tissues you experience the day once you workout. When you workout at most fulfilling tiers, the frame blessings from the motion and techniques the lactic acid effectively and effectively. Just like some thing else, mistaken workout will reason harm; the frame struggles to neutralize the acidity tiers withinside the blood and illness and continual fitness situations are frequently the result.

Over-consumption of stimulants

I get it. You're feeling confused and frazzled and need a bit pick-me-as much as get you aleven though the day, so that you flip to espresso or tea, or maybe cigarettes to offer you that increase which you want. However, these items best serve to get worse your issues and throw your frame into deeper degrees of acidosis. The caffeine in tea and espresso disrupts the stability of your hormones, encouraging the discharge of extra strain hormones into your blood stream. The nicotine in

cigarettes alters the praise facilities withinside the mind and will increase the degrees of the multitude of pollution on your blood stream, ensuing in better acidity, illness and disease.

Medications

Mainstream medicine may be wonderful - it has helped us to conquer many fitness problems and stay higher and longer lives. But it additionally comes with terrible side-results and worse still, those medicinal drugs are acid-forming and pose a extra burden for the frame to should deal with, growing your chance of different illnesses and fitness lawsuits.

It's hardly ever sudden that one of these large percent of the worldwide populace be afflicted by such a lot of fitness situations while you don't forget simply how lots of those acid-forming conduct humans practice. We have become sicker through the 12 months due to the fact we simply deal with the outward signs and don't get to the foundation of the problem.

So, how do you know if a high-level of acidity in your body is the culprit for all of your problems? How can you discover if following an alkaline diet and lifestyle could be your answer? And how can you test your pH levels? Let's find out.

25 Telltale Signs that Your Body is too Acidic

You don't want to be a health practitioner to note the symptoms and symptoms that some thing isn't pretty proper on your frame. You is probably affected by extra sizeable fitness problems along with arthritis or pimples or smaller niggling signs that don't certainly upload as much as much, however are a hard a part of your life. Take coronary heart withinside the reality which you're now no longer alone, and that many different humans have suffered similar to you, best to discover an extraordinary solution.

Here are the top 25 symptoms that suggest that your body is too acidic:

1. Skin lawsuits along with eczema, psoriasis, pimples, hives, dry pores and skin or mysterious rashes that won't clean up.

2. Constant fatigue and mind fog even in case you get the endorsed quantity of sleep every night time.

3. Low mood, depression, and absence of enthusiasm for life.

4. Excess weight, mainly across the waist area.

5. Feeling bloodless whilst others are heat or comfortable.

6. Frequent infections, viruses and different fitness lawsuits.

7. Migraines (mainly with aura) and headaches.

8. Angular cheilitis (cracks on the nook of mouth).

9. Unexplained toothache or mouth pain.

10. Leg cramps and spasms, twitchy legs at night time time.

11. Dull and lank hair with cut up ends. Might shed extra than usual.

12.   Thin nails which are liable to breakage and splitting.

13.   Chronic indigestion and heartburn.

14.   Teeth that chip or smash easily, or are coming lose.

15.   Limbs that sense heavy and absence energy.

16.   Loss of libido.

17.   Hyperactivity, restlessness, elevated sensitivity to noises and sounds.

18.   Mouth ulcers and touchy teeth.

19.   Stomach bloating, trapped wind, diarrhea, illness and different digestive problems.

20.   Pale grey pores and skin.

21.   Insomnia and night time-walking.

22.   Frequent thrush/candida albicans infections.

23.   Cold sores, shingles and different associated herpes flare-ups.

24.   Irregular menstrual cycle and/or trouble conceiving.

25.   Unexplained pores and skin itches or sensitivities to sure kind of fabric.

It's quite probable which you'll be capable of tick off as a minimum one object on that listing there, if now no longer an entire bunch of them. Of course, make certain to seek advice from your health practitioner to talk about your signs so that you can rule out some other underlying fitness problems.

Now, there's a manner you may be extra particular and in reality degree the degrees of acidity on your frame so that you can degree your development as you rework your fitness. This is through checking out your frame's pH degrees. If you're some thing like me, you'll be intrigued through your results - gaining knowledge of approximately your very own frame definitely fascinating. So let's discover the way to do it, shall we?

Testing Your Acidity Levels

There are 3 fundamental methods that you may take a look at the pH stage of your frame. These are blood plasma, urine and saliva.

• Blood plasma trying out gives the maximum correct account of your proper blood pH ranges, however it does have its downsides too. Depending in which withinside the international you are, and whether or not you've got got medical health insurance or now no longer, it could be alternatively high priced and additionally invasive, specially in case you're now no longer too eager on needles. Speak on your practitioner or nearby fitness-trying out health center in case you'd want to understand extra.

• Urine trying out is the following maximum correct manner to check your pH ranges, and is an easy, reasonably-priced manner of trying out from home - you could honestly select out up a percent of pH check strips out of your nearby pharmacy or on line retailer. First factor withinside the morning, get rid of the strip from the percent and both maintain it for your urine stream, or acquire a small quantity in a box to dip the check strip into. The strips extrade colour relying for your pH level, and every colour represents a one-of-a-kind price. Most packs can even consist of a manual on the way to recognize and interpret those consequences. Make certain which you jot down your beginning pH price in a secure region so that you can consult with it at a later date to test your progress. The goal is to have your morning pH degree among 6.five and 7.five.

• Saliva trying out is the least correct technique of all trying out (because the your mouth carries fluctuating ranges of acidic bacteria), however it's also the maximum snug and easy for maximum humans to do. Just as you probably did with the urine check, you could use a pH check strip to degree your saliva's pH level. First, rinse your mouth with water and spit it out, then spit again (and make sure you haven't eaten or brushed your tooth previous to trying out). Collect your saliva onto a spoon and soak the check strip paper. Your consequences must study a pH among
7.0 and 7.5.

Now which you have determined the maximum not unusualplace reasons of a fairly acidic body, the way to pick out the telltale signs and the way to check your pH ranges, we will now flip our cognizance closer to alkalinity and taking our first steps at the route to higher fitness.

The first port of name can be healthful meals, in which we are able to find out scrumptious and fitness-selling vitamins to rebalance your pH ranges. We will then flip our interest to the acid-forming meals which you must lessen out of your day by day eating regimen as plenty as possible. *Now here's a question:* which fruit is fairly acidic however works wonders in alkalizing your body? Find out withinside the subsequent chapter.

CHAPTER 4
Eating For Alkalinity

How wholesome is your eating regimen? Is it as nourishing because it truely should be? Many people consider we're ingesting the first-rate eating regimen we likely can, best to scratch our heads in confusion whilst we nonetheless get sick, be afflicted by low energy, extra weight and depression.

The trouble lies withinside the information. You see, plenty of the nutritional recommendation and fad weight-reduction plan accessible honestly advocates the intake of those acid- forming meals. Societies for the duration of the sector flourish once they comply with their personal conventional diets and forget about what mass advertising is telling them. You best should go searching you to look international ranges of illness and weight problems soar - in element due to following awful nutritional recommendation or the junk-meals epidemic this is spreading from the west. Sadly, it's those sort of inaccurate suggestions that lots of us comply with withinside the quest for maximum fitness, best to go away us questioning why we simply aren't getting higher.

The actual answer is a far less complicated one. Eat an alkalizing eating regimen of LIVE meals and decrease acid forming meals to attain an excellent country of fitness. It truely is simply as easy because it sounds.

Even clinical government are in agreement - for higher typical fitness and an extended life, flip to a plant-wealthy eating regimen. A look at performed at Loma Linda University in California determined that, on average, the ones ingesting this sort of alkalizing eating regimen stay as much as 9.*five years longer than their animal-produce ingesting counterparts.* It's really meals for thought, isn't it?

Everything that crosses our lips creates both acidity or alkalinity inside our our bodies on a various pH scale. The best manner we will surely revel in suitable fitness is to welcome extra scrumptious, alkaline-forming meals, consisting of an abundance of stunning plant meals, inexperienced leafy veggies, culmination, positive nuts and seeds, and flavorsome herbs and spices. Do preserve in thoughts there are positive acid- forming plant meals that must be loved occasionally in case you need the first-rate consequences from this lifestyle. Some entire grains and culmination may be acid forming,

For example, however this doesn't always imply they must be disregarded out of your weight loss plan altogether. Some acid-forming ingredients aren't always 'bad' of their unprocessed shape and nevertheless boast dietary blessings - we simply want to make sure we're eating them withinside the proper stability with the intention to thrive.

Remember to make sure a stability of round 80/20 alkaline to acidic ingredients for satisfactory results. When deciding on to eat acidic ingredients, I endorse choosing extra plant reassets over animal reassets for higher cleansing, nutrients and general fitness. Depending for your circumstances, and with the approval of your healthcare professional, you can of path pick out to base your weight loss plan on 100% alkaline ingredients to faster and extra successfully repair fitness - i.e. you will be feeling rather toxic, stricken by persistent fatigue or low immunity, or combating a debilitating illness.

First up is my listing of fitness-selling ingredients you may absolutely revel in while you are embracing the alkaline lifestyle, observed via way of means of the ones which you must lessen or eliminate. There are many interpretations of the acidic and alkaline meals listing in diverse books and online - a few ingredients are referenced as an acidic AND alkaline meals, so right here I actually have labeled them as satisfactory I can with my personal studies and knowledge. *This listing is supposed as a widespread manual for informational purposes.*

Alkaline Foods

It's an thrilling time of extrade for you, aleven though while we begin a brand new manner of consuming or lifestyle, it's not unusualplace to experience misplaced and uncertain approximately what you may honestly eat. The following precise listing will show to be beneficial if that is the case for you. Everything that looks right here is alkaline-forming and fitness selling.

GREEN LEAFY VEGGIES

Highly alkaline-forming and packed complete of vital vitamins, minerals and phytonutrients in addition to being a extraordinary plant-primarily based totally supply of protein.

These include: Dandelion greens, wild greens, spinach, kale, endive, cabbage, Swiss chard, alfalfa, lettuce, watercress, sea vegetables, seaweed, Pak Choi, escarole, kelp, arugula, collards, mustard greens, spirulina, barley grass, wheatgrass, chlorella.

ROOT VEGGIES

Contain masses of gut-pleasant fiber in an effort to relieve your digestive tract, stability your pH degrees and assist to maintain you feeling satisfied. Also a extraordinary supply of vitamins, minerals and phytonutrients.

These include: Carrots, daikon, potatoes (white, red, yellow and blue), candy potatoes, turnip, swede, beetroot, taro root, parsnip, yams.

OTHER VEGGIES & LEGUMES

Delicious, alkaline-forming, detoxifying and complete of these crucial vitamins.

These include: Fresh inexperienced beans, globe artichokes, bamboo shoots, sprouted beans, cauliflower, broccoli, celery, cucumbers, eggplant, onions, horseradish, kohlrabi, leeks, mushrooms, butternut squash, acorn squash, summer time season squash, candy peppers (red, yellow and inexperienced), cabbage, soybeans (clean, tofu, soy milk), asparagus, pumpkin, radishes, tomato, zucchini, brussels sprouts, string beans, military beans, lima beans, lentils, okra.

FRESH HERBS

Great supply of chlorophyll, a amazing supply of antioxidants, and stocks a number of the identical blessings as inexperienced leafy veggies.

These include: All herbs, inclusive of basil, bay leaf, cilantro (coriander), oregano, dill, marjoram, parsley, sage, candy basil, tarragon, thyme, rosemary and chives.

FRESH FRUITS

Keep your frame satiated, fulfill your candy teeth and maintain your fluid degrees up. Also carries excessive degrees of antioxidants and facilitates sell cleansing and acidity neutralization.

These include: Most end result inclusive of; banana (ripe and spotty), blackberries, grapes (inexperienced and red), peach, persimmon, raspberries, apricot, apple, pear, cherries, cantaloupe melon, water melon, lemon, lime, loganberries, mango, gooseberry, grapefruit, guava, nectarine, oranges, clean figs, peach,

pineapple, rhubarb, strawberries, tangerine, mandarin, satsuma, prickly pear, quince, kiwi fruit, mandarin, tamarind, coconut, sapodilla, blueberries, papaya, rhubarb.

DRIED FRUITS

Incredible supply of iron and a extraordinary addition to recipes that name for that delivered sweetness.

These include: Dates, dried figs, raisins.

HEALTHY FATS

Wholefood fat with fiber and vitamins in tact are higher processed via way of means of the frame while as compared to sophisticated oil. For satisfactory results, revel in moderately and make sure fat aren't the middle of your plate.

These include: Avocados, almonds (almond milk, almond butter), chestnuts, pine nuts, maximum seeds inclusive of sunflower seeds, pumpkin seeds, sesame seeds (tahini), chia seeds, poppy seeds.

CERTAIN GRAINS

Have an alkalizing impact at the frame and are full of vital b- complicated vitamins, minerals and wholesome fiber.

These include: Quinoa, millet, amaranth, wild rice.

SPICES AND SEASONINGS

Contain beneficiant portions of recuperation phytonutrient and compounds, which useful resource withinside the pH stability method, assist your inner organs thru detox, and additionally increase your normal fitness.

These include: All spices, such as chili pepper, cinnamon, curry, ginger, garlic, herbs (all), miso, mustard seed, sea salt, tamari.

MISCELLANEOUS

Highly alkalizing and flexible meals that may be fed on as an addition to a plant-wealthy weight loss plan. Apple cider vinegar is particularly beneficial because it facilitates the frame

to detox and heal.

These include: Fresh fruit and vegetable juices, herbal nevertheless mineral water, umeboshi vinegar, apple cider vinegar, baking soda, blackstrap molasses, stevia, agar, natural teas, tempeh and tofu (now no longer fried), coconut milk, smoothies.

Acidic Foods

We will now flip our interest to the acid-forming meals, which you may lessen or ditch out of your weight loss plan to enhance the manner you think, appearance and sense as a result. The following targeted listing will entail all the meals that create acidity to your frame and may result in terrible fitness and sickness in excess.

PROCESSED SUGARS AND ARTIFICIAL SWEETENERS

The worst offenders in relation to acidity - they feed bacteria, fungus and sickness, location extra strain at the complete frame and appreciably boom the acidification method.

Avoid: White processed sugar, corn syrup, sodas and smooth drinks, fruit jellies, lollies and sweets, processed jams, custards, honey, ketchup, chemical sweeteners, aspartame.

DAIRY PRODUCTS

Highly mucus-forming, stresses the frame, will increase acidity tiers, may also really harm our bones.

Avoid: Cows milk, goat milk, sheep milk, difficult and smooth cheeses, cream, ice cream, yoghurt.

MEAT, FISH AND ANIMAL PRODUCTS

Heavily stresses the frame, such as the digestive system, appreciably disrupts the acid-alkaline stability.

Avoid: Processed meats, beef, carp, clams, cod, corned beef, fish, haddock, lamb, lobster, mussels, organ meats, oyster, pike, pork, rabbit, salmon, sardines, sausage, scallops, shellfish, shrimp, tuna, turkey, veal, venison, eggs.

CERTAIN VEGETABLES

High in sugars and may be acid-forming, aleven though nevertheless boast dietary advantage while eaten in moderation.

Eat occasionally: Corn, wintry weather squash, olives.

CERTAIN FRUITS

Contain acids that aren't as effortlessly metabolised through the frame, that can boom acidity load. Enjoy in moderation.

Avoid: Unripe bananas

Eat occasionally: Plums, damsons, prunes, cranberries, pomegranate.

GRAINS AND GLUTEN PRODUCTS

Contains excessive tiers of the anti-nutrient phytic acid, that is extra tough to digest, binds to calcium, magnesium, zinc and iron and may do away with them from the frame. Gluten may be adverse to the digestive tract.

Avoid: Barley, rye, wheat (aside from wheatgrass and sprouts), gluten-containing spaghetti, pasta, white bread.

Enjoy occasionally: Buckwheat, oats (pick gluten loose), brown rice, white rice, rice milk.

ANIMAL FATS & REFINED OILS

Adhere to the blood cells after consumption, adjust the frame's capacity to detoxify and interferes with the pH stability method.

Avoid: Butter, cream, margarine, animal fats, lard, dripping, canola oil, corn oil, safflower oil.

Omit or use sparingly: Avocado oil, hemp oil, coconut oil, sesame oil, olive oil, flax oil, sunflower oil.

NUTS AND NUT BUTTERS

Contains the anti-nutrient phytic acid, that can prevent the absorption of calcium, magnesium, iron and zinc. Enjoy in moderation.

Eat occasionally: Brazil nuts, cashews, pecans, pistachios, hazelnuts, macadamia nuts, walnuts, peanuts.

ALCOHOL

A toxin that locations greater stress at the frame, hinders the pH neutralization method and is notably acidic. Increases belly acid.

Avoid: Wine, beer, spirits, liquor.

CAFFEINE

Places stress at the frame's hormonal structures and disrupts pH stability as a result. Over-stimulates the strain hormones and will increase pollution withinside the frame.

Avoid: Black tea, coffee, electricity drinks, caffeine capsules or stimulants.

Enjoy occasionally: Green tea, dairy loose darkish chocolate, cocoa and dairy loose warm chocolate drinks.

LEGUMES

Contain anti-nutrient phytic acid, that can intrude with the absorption of nutrients, aleven though nevertheless boast dietary advantage while eaten in moderation.

Avoid: Fried tofu.

Eat occasionally: Black beans, chickpeas, inexperienced peas, kidney beans, pinto beans, purple beans, white beans.

JUNK/PROCESSED FOOD

Places extra stress at the body, interfering with cleansing processes, feeds bacteria, disease, fungus and candida, piles at the weight, specifically with out vitamins but excessive in processed sugars and fats.

Avoid: Biscuits, cakes, pastries, fried ingredients, burgers, takeaway ingredients, desk salt, fries, 'heath' bars, chips, processed meats, sodas and tender liquids consisting of colas.

The Uncertain Foods

There are positive ingredients that many are nonetheless uncertain of in phrases of alkalinity. Some of those ingredients have already been categorised withinside the preceding lists, aleven though they're really well worth bringing up once more as they purpose a lot war of words among individuals who observe an alkaline weight loss program and life-style. Use your discretion with those ingredients, and don't forget that we're aiming for an 80/20 ratio. You do not want to stick strictly to alkaline ingredients, so that you can experience those ingredients inside stability ought to you wish.

These include:

Brazil nuts, buckwheat, cashews, flax seeds, kombucha, quinoa, fermented veggies (sauerkraut), soy merchandise, maple syrup, blueberries, tomatoes, corn, flax seeds, inexperienced tea, pumpkin seeds, sunflower seeds, white potatoes.

Did you figure out the solution to the query I requested you on the quit of the remaining chapter?
What is a exceedingly acidic fruit that may be a powerful alkalizing agent while consumed?

You bet it - lemon. This citrus fruit is excellent in your body, and I exceedingly endorse consuming the juice of 1/2 of a lemon in a tumbler of water first aspect every morning. The identical may be stated for all styles of citrus fruit, so experience them as you wish.

Extra Dietary Tips to Boost Alkalinity:

• Drink lemon water upon rising, first aspect every morning (or a sprint of apple cider vinegar in water)

• Drink sufficient spring water (or on the least, filtered water) during the day

• Emphasize stay plant ingredients

• Incorporate inexperienced powders into your juices and smoothies, consisting of wheatgrass or barley grass

• Regularly devour baking soda (sodium bicarbonate), aleven though now no longer with meals as it could intervene with digestion and belly acids. *See measurements* *for a simple baking soda tonic in the <u>recipe section</u>.*

• Replace your espresso dependancy with natural tea

• Choose sea salt over acid-forming desk salt

• Many condiments are exceedingly acidic (consisting of ketchup, processed mustards and mayonnaise), so maintain those to a minimal and strive developing your personal wholesome sauces and toppings from complete-ingredients

• Use apple cider vinegar or citrus in salad dressings

• Choose clean greens over canned, pickled or frozen

• Choose natural produce in which possible, as insecticides can compromises a number of the alkalizing results of the meals

• Replace gluten-containing pasta with pasta crafted from quinoa, or choose complete quinoa, wild rice or millet instead

• If the use of sweeteners, ditch the synthetic stuff and pick greater herbal merchandise consisting of stevia, coconut sugar or maple sugar

• Arm your self with some go-to alkaline food to make sure you don't fall off plan (there are a gaggle of alkaline recipes online, plus the scrumptious beverage recipes on the quit of this book)

• Because many alkaline ingredients are certainly decrease in energy in assessment to acidic ingredients, make sure you consume sufficient. Under consuming can set you up for failure in this life-style - do now no longer limition your energy. You can middle your plate round satisfying, filling ingredients (consisting of candy potatoes and root greens) with beneficiant servings of vegetables and different healthful alkaline ingredients to gas you with energy.

Now it's time to transport on from dietery subjects and check natural treatments and wholesome life-style conduct that you could use to rebalance your pH ranges and sense excellent. This consists of herbs, spices, dietary supplements and sleep, which we can cowl withinside the subsequent chapter.

CHAPTER 5

Herbal Healing and Lifestyle Tips

Healing is set some distance greater than simply concentrated on a set of signs and hoping that your sickness will clean up. Even if this indicates a entire overhaul of your weight loss program and clearing out all the junk and changing it with healthful alkaline ingredients.

Of course, you maximum virtually will see excellent outcomes to your hair, skin, vitality, average fitness and readability of concept with the aid of using consuming clean, however this isn't the entire picture. Your weight loss program isn't the handiest purpose of excessive acidity status, and there are different matters to blame, consisting of your surroundings and the life-style selections which you make.

Western medication has an inclination to peer every frame element as break away the whole, and as a end result frequently fails to get results. The key's to deal with the frame holistically, the usage of diet, way of life, environment, and opportunity treatments to heal the whole frame - getting proper right all the way down to the foundation of the problem, fixing the fitness difficulty this is bothering you the maximum, and frequently clearing many others on the identical time.

This bankruptcy is devoted to simply that. Here we can first delve deeper into opportunity treatments which might be to be had to you, from ordinary herbs and spices to rebalancing and recuperation dietary supplements. We will then awareness at the easy but powerful way of life conduct that you could undertake speedy and without problems from the consolation of your personal home, after which we can carry all of it collectively with the aid of using searching at the way to get commenced, inclusive of a few worthwhile guidelines that my friend, Maria, taught me to make the procedure easier. Let's get commenced with natural recuperation.

Herbs, Spices and Supplements

If you're searching out a herbal and powerful manner to rebalance your pH degrees and increase your recuperation procedure, herbs, spices and dietary supplements are a powerful

option. Herbs and spices are smooth to find, cheaper to buy, and now no longer to say scrumptious too!

Within this phase you may discover a big form of treatments for informational purposes. Knowledge is power - honestly take a while to get familiar with every method to make an knowledgeable choice as to what is going to paintings nice for you and your circumstances. You might also additionally need to awareness on some or maybe simply one treatment at a time. Never hesitate to talk about the country of your fitness together along with your healthcare practitioner to decide which dietary supplements are maximum proper in your circumstances. Always use herbs and dietary supplements in a cautious, knowledgeable manner.

Herbs

Herb are nature's powerhouses, packed complete of fitness-giving vitamins, minerals, phytonutrients and antioxidants to assist to nourish your frame, heal ailment, save you the onset of sure ailments and additionally rebalance that all- crucial pH level.

Culinary herbs

Culinary herbs are the perfect to advantage from as you could upload them to nearly any form of dish for brought taste and nutrients. And they don't should price you something either - you could develop your personal aromatic herb garden (exterior or maybe to your windowsill) to revel in them as frequently as you like. Choose from herbs like basil, bay leaf, cilantro (coriander), oregano, dill, marjoram, parsley, sage, candy basil, tarragon, thyme, rosemary, or some other inexperienced leafy herbs you would possibly have to be had.

Herbal Teas

You also can drink an array of natural teas at the alkaline way of life, consisting of peppermint, chamomile, rose hip, rooibos and licorice - all of which can be first-rate manner to cleanse and detox your frame, hold you hydrated, and upload a dietary increase in your diet. Herbal teas can assist to rebalance your pH and additionally deal with any signs and symptoms of acidity you is probably struggling from, inclusive of anxiety, depression, insomnia, digestive issues, IBS, indigestion and migraines. A first-rate replacement for the instances you're craving a cup of some thing heat and soothing, however ordinary tea and espresso is off the menu.

There are also many medicinal herbs that you can enjoy in tablet,

capsule, tea or tincture form. *These include:*

• *Dandelion and Burdock*

Both of those herbs are fantastically alkalizing and assist to purify the blood and liver.

• *Black Cohosh*

Black cohosh is widely recognized for assisting to stability the frame's endocrine system, in addition to cleaning the colon, liver and kidneys even as alkalizing your system.

• *Slippery Elm Bark*

Slippery elm is nice referred to as a remedy for irritation and belly and digestive ailments, however also can stability your pH degrees and cleanse your blood.

• *Devils Claw*

Devil's claw is a top notch treatment to assist to sell alkalinity and decrease the degrees of candida albicans withinside the system - the yeast that frequently reasons a large number of infections and pores and skin conditions.

• *Sarsaparilla*

If you're bothered with any pores and skin conditions, then sarsaparilla would possibly simply be your answer. Not most effective does it assist to rebalance your pH degrees, it additionally purifies the blood and has an antibacterial and anti inflammatory action.

Spices

Spices are certainly considered one among nature's marvel drugs. They provide the identical form of nutrients, phytonutrients and antioxidants as wholefoods and herbs do, however additionally they comprise a large number of strong ailment preventing compounds to assist heal your frame and save you sick fitness. *Here are the a number of the handiest ones:*

Cumin

This spice is not unusualplace in maximum ethnic cuisines and is definitely scrumptious. It has a robust alkalizing impact at the frame, and also can address digestive signs and symptoms consisting of flatulence, diarrhea and

IBS.

Turmeric

Turmeric is the spice that offers curry its yellow color. It's filled with an antioxidant known as curcumin, which has been used to assist deal with of some of fitness problems inclusive of cancers, Alzheimer's disorder and inflammatory conditions - in addition to boosting your mind feature, happiness and memory. It has a effective pH balancing impact at the frame and must be covered to your eating regimen each day.

Cayenne

Cayenne pepper is one of the maximum alkalizing spices known. It works wonders at the endocrine device and has powerful anti-oxidant qualities, making it a precious all-rounder for excellent fitness. Beware though - it is able to be hot!

Ginger

Ginger is a excellent addition to any alkalizing eating regimen, as it's far a powerful cleanser, anti- illness treatment and tastes scrumptious too. You can revel in it in tea shape, pill shape, or delivered in your favourite dish.

Fennel

With its wealthy aniseed taste and fragrance, fennel is rather soothing at the digestive device, excessive in antioxidants (which facilitates guard the frame from disorder) and is packed complete of minerals like iron, copper, potassium and calcium. Enjoy it as a tea or delivered in your meals.

Last however now no longer least, let's test which dietary supplements can rebalance your pH ranges.

Supplements

Supplements can assist kick-begin the restoration method through filling any dietary holes which have happened from bad digestion or a beyond of nutritional unbalance.

Some of those dietary supplements are important (you'll discover why in a moment) and lots of have a powerful alkalizing impact at the frame. Feel unfastened to talk about any of those alternatives together along with your healthcare practitioner to make certain they're appropriate for you.

Calcium

You would possibly consider from our in advance chapters that after your frame struggles to neutralize a excessive stage of acidity, it steals minerals like calcium and magnesium out of your bones to assist it attempt to cope. This leaves our bones susceptible and susceptible to osteoporosis and standard damage, which we want to save you earlier than it's too late. It's encouraged which you take a tremendous calcium complement whilst you transition to an alkaline eating regimen so that you can update the ones minerals which you misplaced out of your bones, and additionally make certain you are becoming sufficient diet D from herbal daylight to reinforce calcium's absorption.

Choose a good emblem of calcium dietary supplements, and intention for among 800 to 1500mg according to day. Plenty of leafy veggies also are a excellent manner to get to your each day calcium intake.

Magnesium

Magnesium is any other mineral this is used to fight excessive ranges of acidity withinside the frame. It's additionally the mineral that a big percent of the populace is poor in, so it's vital to take a complement or take everyday Epsom salt baths to take in this important mineral. Magnesium is likewise vital for mind feature and may alleviate migraines, anxiety complications and hormonal imbalances in women. Take 400-800mg according to day, ideally with meals.

Almonds also are a exceptional whole-meals supply of magnesium.

If you are interested in learning more about Epsom salt, you may also benefit from my book: _Epsom Salt: 50 Miraculous Benefits, Uses & Natural Remedies for Your Health, Body & Home_.

Kelp

Traditionally, kelp has been taken in complement shape as a dense supply of antioxidants and nutrients. It's a kind of seaweed that includes excessive ranges of iodine (for thyroid feature), magnesium, and additionally has powerful detoxifying and alkalizing consequences upon the frame. It's very cheaper and may be observed in pill, pill and tincture shape a maximum fitness-meals stores. Follow the dosage

suggestions at the label. You may even purchase kelp withinside the shape of noodles (a excellent manner to update gluten pasta) or in a shaker to feature a sprinkle of taste your meals.

Chlorella

Chlorella is a kind of algae this is excessive in wholesome protein, nutrients and minerals and additionally acts as a powerful detoxifier and alkalizing agent. It's additionally powerful in boosting the immune device and preventing off infection (a not unsualplace end result of acidity), in addition to selling exact intestine bacteria. It's without difficulty observed in maximum fitness meals stores in pill or pill shape. Again, comply with the dosage commands at the packaging.

Spirulina

Like kelp and chlorella, spirulina (additionally a sort of algae) is a mighty supply of minerals, antioxidants and amino acids which are located in inexperienced leafy greens - so that you can get maximum of the advantages that inexperienced leafy greens offer, specifically in case you're now no longer this kind of big fan of ingesting greens. It's a exceptional manner to soak up your omega-6 and omega-three fatty acids while balancing your pH on the identical time. You can locate it in pill or tablet shape, and additionally in electricity shape in lots of fitness meals stores. Follow the dosage pointers at the label.

You can revel in those awesome herbs, spices and dietary supplements on a every day foundation to help you in your restoration adventure - and to offer you a touch head- start. You will assist restore the harm inflicted via way of means of years of acidity, deal with the symptoms, rebalance your pH tiers and additionally enhance your nutrition.

Next, let's test the easy life-style guidelines that may similarly assist you on your adventure to alkalinity!

Lifestyle Tips

As noted earlier, your typical life-style performs a giant function on your fitness status, and specifically so in relation to the pH stability inside your frame. There are such a lot of life-style conduct and demanding situations that may provide upward thrust to excessive tiers of acidity in the frame, so it's simply as essential that we expand new wholesome life-style conduct to help alkalinity together with ingesting the proper foods. In this phase I will percentage with you 7 effective life-style guidelines
on the way to help in balancing your frame's pH value.

Tip #1: Manage stress

Most folks are below a diploma of strain each unmarried day of our lives -

there's truely no manner of averting it withinside the cutting-edge age. A positive quantity of strain is certainly a healthful factor via way of means of supporting us the texture each challenged and motivated, however while tiers of strain grow to be chronic, they positioned the frame below high-quality quantities of stress and reason a extreme acid/alkaline unbalance in addition to inflicting many different fitness problems.

Stress reasons your digestive gadget to close down, which then limits the vitamins that your frame is capable of absorb (leaving your extra susceptible than ever to unwell fitness). And now no longer handiest that, however strain additionally disrupts your hormones; growing the strain hormone cortisol and growing tiers of unfastened radicals which could result in cell harm, dementia, coronary heart sickness or even cancers.

As you could imagine, it's very essential which you take steps to manipulate your strain tiers and additionally analyze powerful strain-control strategies so that you can move directly to stay your ordinary existence with out poor aftereffects. Firstly, recall if there's a manner you could lessen the extent of strain you're below. This would possibly suggest delegating essential obligations to the ones round you, taking day out for your self, or maybe saying 'no' each as soon as in a while.

Then recall which strain-control strategies might great accommodate your life-style. There are many obtainable so take a while to locate one which works for you. My private favorites consist of yoga, meditation and tai chi, and I'm great capable of disconnect and recharge once I locate solace in my yoga practice. What might be your favored practice?

Tip #2: Breathe

Do you recognize a way to breathe properly? We've all been doing it because the day we have been born, however a lot of us expand awful conduct and handiest get a small percent of the oxygen that we want to feed our tissues and our brain, make sure our metabolic approaches paintings effectively and additionally keep a healthful alkaline frame. In fact, accurate respiration is most of the maximum alkalizing practices there's obtainable. Best of all, it's honestly unfastened and it's going to make you experience calmer and happier too.

So learn how to breathe effectively via way of means of attempting this easy exercise:

1) Breathe in for two counts, filling the decrease a part of your lung first, then the center, then the higher part.

2) Hold this breath for a remember of 8. It would possibly experience tricky, however hold in there - it'll get easier.

3) Slowly breathe out for four counts, first emptying the higher a part of your lungs, then the center then the decrease.

4) Then repeat the cycle 10 times.

Tip #3: Sleep

I've been advised that Elle MacPherson's favored a part of the alkaline life-style is permitting herself the more sleep she so desires, and I couldn't accept as true with her extra. Sleep is your frame's manner of repairing broken tissues, restoration, developing and additionally rebalancing the endocrine gadget and pH stability - so in case you aren't getting your premiere stage of sleep, you aren't doing your self any favors and retaining your frame in a unwell acidic state.

So, make it your precedence to sleep! Write it to your diary withinside the identical manner as you will some other vital appointment and keep on with it. You owe it to yourself. Aim to get round 8 hours of sleep in line with night. Of course, your most suitable stage will range relying to your personal non-public needs.

Tip #4: Stay hydrated and switch your drinking water

We all recognise that staying hydrated is vital, however how secure is your faucet water? In many nations and areas across the globe, faucet water includes contaminants and acid-forming chemicals, which over the years can slowly harm our fitness. Did you understand that really switching your ingesting water could make a big distinction in your fitness and electricity tiers? It is stated that the handiest manner to alkalize water is with a water ionizer machine, which produces water with a pH that you could choose, and filters the water of toxins, metals and sediments. This can but pose as an steeply-priced alternative for some, so I really endorse deciding on spring water wherein possible

(maintain in thoughts that quite a few bottled water is largely faucet water, so study labels), or on the least, drink filtered faucet water (counter pinnacle or below counter water filters) to cast off as many sediments and contaminants as possible. Whatever your alternatives are, it's far continually extraordinarily vital to live hydrated, even though faucet water is your most effective choice!

Tip #5: Get more exercise

Physical pastime is essential for the human frame as all of us recognise. Many folks stay sedentary lifestyles, shifting from mendacity in bed, to sitting in our cars, at our desks, then returning domestic to flop at the sofa. Rinse. Repeat. All it takes is shifting greater. Walk to the neighborhood shop in place of driving, recollect taking a dance magnificence or playing your preferred recreation on a greater ordinary basis. Take up running, or walking, or some thing else you fancy. What should you do nowadays to get shifting?

Tip #6: Quit birth control and HRT

Synthetic hormones are horrific news, something your age. Not most effective are they extraordinarily poisonous in your whole frame and tremendously acid-forming, additionally they mess together along with your endocrine gadget, developing synthetic situations which most effective extend your struggling and disrupt your frame's herbal balance. There are many different gentler alternatives obtainable in keeping off undesirable pregnancies, surviving your menopausal signs and treating your pimples than consuming synthetic hormones. To learn more about holistic remedies in treating various hormonal issues, you can advantage from my bestseller: *Herbal Hormone Handbook*.

Tip #7: Avoid plastic

It may appear to be an harmless act to shop for meals from plastic containers, to shop your leftovers in plastic bins and to drink from plastic water bottles, however through doing so we're virtually disrupting our pH tiers and inflicting all types of nasty fitness problems. You see; plastic virtually mimics estrogen, additionally interfering together along with your endocrine gadget and developing havoc, illness and acidity. The exceptional alternative is to update as a number of the plastics in your private home with options including glass or stainless steel, which includes water bottles, lunch bins and garage bins.

By following those easy way of life hints, you take a big step closer to restoration your frame and rebalancing your pH balance. And now no longer simply that, your intellectual fitness and happiness can even improve, which in itself could have a vast impact upon your confidence.

We've nearly reached the give up of this ee-e book and also you ought to be feeling stimulated and inspired to make those vital adjustments to your lifestyles to peer your fitness, happiness and typical health soar. But first, I'd want to percentage with you the maximum vital hints and hints which you want to recognise whilst you start off in this adventure so you are installation for success, now no longer failure. Let's take a look.

Extra Tips and Tricks To Help Your Journey

Despite exceptional intentions, many humans really fail while they are trying to undertake a modern weight-reduction plan or way of life and it's now no longer absolutely their fault. They throw themselves 100% into new behavior with out in search of the recommendation or assist of others, suffering to resist their antique cravings, or maybe dropping the incentive once they haven't speedy misplaced the ones twenty kilos or cleared up their pimples withinside the identical week. It's no surprise that such a lot of humans fail withinside the first few days.

Let's get matters clear, the alkaline weight-reduction plan and way of life is never tough or difficult - particularly in case you make certain you're ingesting enough (remember, your quantities of alkaline meals will want to be large than you is probably used to), however your mind-set and expectancies could make this revel in difficult in case you permit them. Without the assist and recommendation of a depended on friend, you can fail earlier than you even get started.

I became one of the fortunate ones. When I witnessed Maria's superb transformation and commenced my very own journey, I already had all the assist and aid I should ask for. Her suggestions and aid supposed that I should slip into the alkaline eating regimen distinctly effortlessly and most significantly stick with it on a long-time period foundation to make sure that I didn't simply get wholesome, I additionally stayed wholesome.

And that is precisely what I'm going to do for you. The following suggestions are tried- and-examined and could make a large distinction for your success.

Take it slow

I apprehend you're feeling pumped and captivated with reworking your existence and also you need to get consequences overnight. So you throw your self in and do clearly the entirety to the letter. I congratulate you - in no way lose that enthusiasm and power to reap higher fitness! But, and it's a massive however, you is probably making the adventure closer to restoration a good deal more difficult than it desires to be.

Drastic modifications are frequently now no longer sustainable. Not simplest are you much more likely to provide in and consume that ill-inflicting sweet or steak, you're additionally much more likely to bodily go through as a end result as your frame starts to cleanse the pollution it has accumulated, then manner and put off them.

So instead, make small modifications as you cross. Try a tweak right here and a tweak there to get commenced, then retain to feature extra fitness-giving practices on a day by day or weekly foundation to fit your needs and your way of life. For example, you may determine that this week you may introduce extra plant meals into your eating regimen, and update your everyday dairy yoghurt with soya or coconut yoghurt instead.
That's an wonderful first step to take and one so one can shape a firm (and with any luck lasting) basis to the relaxation.

Then pick out your subsequent step - possibly changing meat with protein-wealthy legumes, or swapping dairy milk with almond milk, or attempting wild rice in place of white pasta - and retain till you've got got reached the whole alkaline eating regimen ideal. It's no quick-repair however it'll create lasting change.

Expect Detox Symptoms

From the very second you begin to make wholesome modifications and undertake an alkaline eating regimen and way of life, your fitness will improve. Your bones will fill with the critical minerals that acidity has stolen, candida albicans will slowly disappear, oxygen will fill your each mobileular and your kidneys, liver, lungs and pores and skin will paintings difficult to put off the ones pollution that made you unwell and obese withinside the first place. Think of it like a huge spring easy - there's going to be a piece of untidiness as you clean out, you may want to get your fingers dirty, however the end result can be a colourful and glowing you.

So of path you're pretty possibly to revel in a few detox signs and symptoms as the
spring easy is going on. Such as headaches (in particular from caffeine withdrawal), belly troubles and bloating, antique meals cravings, low strength stages, pores and skin breakouts and irritability. Don't be overly involved approximately those signs and symptoms - they're only brief and

also you'll quickly have sparkling pores and skin, superb strength stages and freedom from fitness troubles.

But for now, cross clean on your self. Clear your calendar of disturbing obligations, get masses of relaxation and relaxation, get a few sparkling air, experience early nights and you'll quickly experience higher. There's additionally simply a threat which you is probably one of the fortunate ones and bypass this step altogether, in particular when you have a pretty easy, plant-wealthy eating regimen already. Lucky you!

Get a Support System

Don't attempt to cross it alone - get your self a aid machine who will pay attention for your issues and proceedings and assist you get thru any demanding situations you may encounter, consisting of a near buddy or own circle of relatives member. I clearly can't pressure its significance sufficient. Of path, it's quality to pick out someone this is fascinated or sympathetic for your way of life and can be there whilst you want them the most. Who knows, you may even train and encourage them sufficient to sign up for you too!

Be patient

When you undertake an alkaline way of life and eating regimen, it's proper that your frame right away modifications and your pH stability starts to transport closer to a extra regular level. However, for the whole consequences, it's going to take time. Don't assume to awaken the subsequent morning miraculously cured out of your fitness proceedings, searching slimmer and more youthful and extra energetic. You and I each realize that it doesn't paintings like that, and absolutely everyone who indicates that it does is suspect. *Healing takes time - simple and simple.*

The alkaline weight-reduction plan and way of life is a long-time period approach to higher fitness and vibrancy. It's no quick-repair that you may undertake and drop while you sense like it, it's now no longer every other fad yo-yo weight-reduction plan a good way to disappoint. It's a holistic method to higher fitness that takes time. It took your frame a few years or maybe a long time to attain its modern country of sickness, and it'll take greater than an afternoon to go back to complete fitness one again. Balance takes time, however it'll happen, and the results
are really well worth it!

When you begin your adventure closer to an alkaline weight-reduction plan, endure these items in mind. Take it slowly, assume detox symptoms, get a pal on board and be patient. You may be surprised at your transformation!

CHAPTER 1

Alkalizing Fresh Juice Recipes

Your day by day multivitamin has in no way tasted higher. Fresh juices provide a myriad of fitness blessings, and are a good deal greater advanced to the low nutrient, preserved juices out of your supermarket.

It's critical for fitness to live optimally hydrated, and those juices will assist you do simply that, plus greater. Because juicing eliminates fibre from culmination and vegetables, it's miles a splendid manner that will help you soak up and obtain focused nutrients with much less digestive effort. Juices are complete of important electrolytes, phytochemicals, nutrients and minerals - are exceptionally alkalizing, complete of antioxidants, and a remarkable manner to % in a few extra veggies while not having to chunk your manner thru kilos of the stuff.

For most flavor and fitness blessings, it's miles high-quality to drink juices inside thirty mins of being made - aleven though if you're in a pinch, you may location juices in an hermetic field to keep away from oxidization (glass jars paintings remarkable) and shop withinside the refrigerator.

Here are 5 of my favourite juice recipes that I revel in frequently to preserve my frame alkalized. Enjoy!

Beet, Carrot & Ginger Zinger

Beetroot is an notable alkalizing agent, a remarkable blood cleaner and a mighty supply of antioxidant and phytonutrients. The addition of lemon boosts its alkalizing powers, and ginger provides a cleansing, zingy kick.

Ingredients

- 3 medium beets
- 2 large carrots

- 1 lemon
- 1 inch piece of fresh ginger
- 2 green apples, preferably golden delicious or granny smith variety.

Method

1. Carefully peel the beets to keep away from them tasting bitter.

2. Chop carrots and apples, and peel lemon to keep away from bitterness.

3. Press all substances thru your juicer, along side the small piece of ginger.

4. Juice and revel in!

Refreshing Mint & Apple Green-Blitz

An apple an afternoon genuinely does preserve the health practitioner away. Apples are exceptionally alkalizing, comprise most cancers-preventing phytonutrients and additionally upload a scrumptious observe of sweetness to any juice. Add them to hydrating cucumber, anti-oxidant packed kale, clean mint and alkalizing lemon, and you've your self a mild and clean recipe for top notch fitness.

Ingredients

- 2 medium cucumbers
- Small handful of fresh mint
- 6 kale leaves (or alternatively, a small handful of spinach)
- 1 lemon
- 2 green apples, preferably golden delicious or granny smith variety.

Method

1. Peel the lemon and cut up your apples and veggies.

2. Press all substances thru your juicer.

3. Juice and revel in!

Minimalist Melon & Lemon Wonder

This is certainly considered one among my go-to recipes after I need some thing smooth and energizing. It's simple, candy and completely scrumptious. Watermelon and lemon are each exceptionally alkalizing and comprise excessive stages of diet C, antioxidants, phytonutrients and additionally enzymes which assist to preserve your hormones in balance.

Ingredients

- Watermelon, 2 cups

- ½ lemon, peeled

- Mint to garnish (optional)

Method

1. Chop and de-seed watermelon and press thru your juicer, along side lemon.

2. Juice, garnish and revel in!

Alkalizing Berry Detox Juice

This juice packs a actual punch withinside the nutrients stakes, loaded with critical nutrients, minerals, antioxidants and phytonutrients and is exceptionally alkalizing to your frame. And the blessings don't simply prevent there. Raspberries comprise a compound referred to as ellagic acid, which allows save you most cancers and aids healing whilst the frame is recovery from any form of disease. Strawberries additionally assist detoxify the frame, sooth the digestive gadget and are exceptionally alkalizing.

Ingredients

- 2 medium green apples, preferably golden delicious or granny smith varieties.
- 1 handful fresh raspberries
- 1 handful fresh strawberries
- ½ lemon

Method

1. Chop apples and peel the lemon.

2. Press them thru your juicer, along side the raspberries and strawberries (you may go away the strawberry tops on for added minerals).

3. Juice and revel in!

Orange, Sweet Potato & Lime Creamsicle

Carrots are a terrifi supply of antioxidants and diet A - they're very alkalizing and detoxifying at the frame and are remarkable for eye and mind function. Sweet potatoes would possibly appear like a odd aspect for juicing, however you'll be pleasantly amazed with the aid of using their diffused creaminess and dessert-like flavor (now no longer to say their alkalizing blessings). Add a few zesty citrus juices and you've a scrumptious mixture that you'll be addicted to!

Ingredients

- 4 fresh carrots, ends trimmed
- 1 raw medium sweet potato, peeled
- 2 medium oranges
- 1 lime

Method

1. Peel the oranges, lime and candy potato. Top and tail the carrots.

2. Add all the substances on your juicer.

3. Juice (stress if necessary) and revel in!

CHAPTER 2

Deliciously Alkalizing Smoothie Recipes

Alkalizing smoothies are a brief and clean manner to fill your tummy and % in as many wholesome clean fruit and vegetables as you may. They make the best breakfast or gratifying snack for whilst starvation hits in the course of the day.

They're complete of soluble plant fiber which advantages your complete digestive machine, they maintain you feeling glad and assist to combat unfastened-radicals, in addition to imparting endless advantages withinside the manner of vitamins, minerals, phytonutrients and recuperation compounds.

Consider whipping up a big batch withinside the morning, pouring it right into a stainless-steel bottle, and taking with you to revel in in the course of the day - there's much less want to fear approximately deterioration than with juices. Although they usually flavor higher clean, they nevertheless flavor tremendous after an hour or two.

You'll observe that each one of the recipes on this ee-e book are sincerely inexperienced smoothies. This is due to the fact vegetables are, with out doubt, one the exceptional meals picks you may make in relation to returning your frame to its best pH levels. Don't permit this difficulty you though - those combos flavor honestly scrumptious. Feel unfastened to lower or boom the quantities of vegetables you operate in step with your preference. You may turn to the *Alkaline Foods* section in the main *Alkaline Diet* book to get more ideas of the kind of green leafy veggies or fruits you can enjoy in your alkalizing smoothies.

Here are my pass-to recipes once I want some thing filling, alkalizing and nutritious. Hope you want them!

Cleansing Summer Berry Smoothie

If you're eager to begin inclusive of greater vegetables for your smoothies however aren't too positive the way to get started, this recipe is best for you. It consists of juicy berries, creamy banana, gentle spinach leaves and tangy lemon juice to create a scrumptious vitamin, mineral and antioxidant packed feast.

Ingredients

- 1 ripe banana (or more if hungry)

- 1 cup (140g approx.) blackberries, raspberries or strawberries, fresh or frozen

- Handful fresh baby spinach

- Juice of ½ lemon

Method

1. Blend the infant spinach leaves in a small quantity of water

2. Peel your banana and upload to the spinach for your blender, and additionally the relaxation of the components.

3. Blend till easy and creamy.

4. Enjoy!

Peach & Coconut Heaven Smoothie

Want to pattern heaven in a glass? You won't pass a ways incorrect with this tropical treat. It's some other tasty recipe this is tremendous for inexperienced smoothie beginners and additionally gives the distinctly alkalizing powers of coconut water, which gives important electrolytes and enables preserve powerful hydration, and ripe juicy peach, which gives extremely good quantities of vitamins and phytochemicals.

Ingredients

- 1 ripe peach

- 1 ripe banana

- 6 kale leaves (without spines)

- 1 cup (250ml) coconut water

Method

1. Pour the coconut water into your blender. Add the kale and mix till easy.

2. Next peel the banana and de-stone the peach.

3. In your blender, upload the fruit to the spinach-coconut water aggregate and blitz till easy.

4. Enjoy!

Healing Cherry & Basil Smoothie

Ever heard approximately the advantages of basil for the frame? Not most effective is it exceedingly alkalizing and excessive in fitness-improving chlorophyll, it additionally successfully relieves stress, boosts your immune machine and has a robust anti- inflammatory action. Team this with the alkalizing strength of lime juice, electrolyte-packed coconut water and anti-aging, melatonin-wealthy cherries, and you've your self a real superfood smoothie. Yum!

Ingredients

- 1 cup frozen cherries

- Juice of 1 lime

- 1 cup (250ml) coconut water
- Generous handful of basil leaves

Method

1. Pour coconut water into your blender, upload basil and mix till easy.

2. Add to this the cherries and lime juice.

3. Blend till easy and revel in!

Spiced Melon and Fig Smoothie

This recipe turned into located pretty through risk as I experimented in my kitchen one day, and I'm positive you'll agree that the taste is honestly delightful.

Melon is outstanding hydrating, fig is exceedingly alkalizing and aids each cleansing and pH balance, spinach packs a further inexperienced nutrient punch and the cinnamon provides a pleasantly highly spiced surprise - its energetic ingredient, cinnamaldehyde, gives a large number of fitness advantages, inclusive of balancing your pH levels, handling your blood-sugar levels, protects in opposition to most cancers and disorder and gives an antioxidant improve too.

Ingredients

- 2 cups cantaloupe, cubed
- 3 figs (either fresh or dried and soaked in a bowl of warm water).
- 3 cups fresh baby spinach
- 1 medium mango
- ½ teaspoon ground cinnamon

Method

1. First area the melon for your blender and mix till easy. Then

upload the spinach and mix again.

2. Next peel and de-stone the mango.

3. Add the mango to the blender together with the relaxation of the components and mix till easy and creamy.

4. Enjoy!

Tropical Green Herbal Smoothie

Who'd have concept that herbs may want to paintings so nicely in a smoothie? This precise recipe is filled with mango and pineapple which provide a gaggle of vitamins, minerals, antioxidants and tropical taste - then we take it to an entire new stage with the aid of using including veggies and herbs which upload a specific be aware of the Mediterranean, are health-boosting, cleansing, include pH balancing chlorophyll, and masses greater recuperation phytochemicals. You'll open up an entire new international of taste while you attempt natural smoothies.

Ingredients

- 1 mango
- 2 cups pineapple, cubed
- 4 medium stalks of celery
- 1 cup fresh baby spinach
- 1 cup fresh flat-leaf parsley
- ½ cup fresh arugula (rocket)
- ½ teaspoon fresh rosemary

Method

1. Firstly, kind of chop the child spinach, flat-leaf parsley, arugula and rosemary and location withinside the blender.

2. Add a small quantity of filtered water and mix till smooth.

3. Next, get rid of the veins from the celery, de-stone and chop

the mango and peel and slice the pineapple.

4. Throw all of those substances into your blender with the veggies and mix till smooth. Add greater water if wished.
5. Enjoy!

CHAPTER 3

Powerful Teas & Tonics

Everyone loves ingesting tea in my family, particularly me. So after I began out following the alkaline lifestyle, I quickly realised that I desperately wished some thing to update my tea ingesting habit, and a soggy bag of bland chamomile tea simply wasn't going to reduce it. Enter the 'DIY brew' mission!

After a ton of experimentation and countless sampling sessions (a lot to the pleasure of my friends!) I created a few drinks which might be a scrumptious replacement for tea and coffee, % in masses of greater vitamins and recuperation compounds and additionally assist to stability your pH degrees. The end result is scrumptious, healthy, refreshing, and best for any time of the day. All of the tea recipes may be loved both warm or cold, relying for your preference. Make a massive jug of the stuff and sip every time you please.

I'll additionally consist of 3 first-rate recipes for alkalizing tonics, which might be best for the ones instances you simply need the blessings with none fuss. Enjoy!

Perfect Peach & Mint Iced Tea

If you're searching out a tea with a twist, then you've come to the proper location. Jazz up soothing mint tea with a dose of peach and citrus, and you've a flavor sensation so one can stability your pH degrees, sell an alkaline frame and assist you sense first-rate - and is filled with vital vitamins, minerals and antioxidants.

Ingredients

- 4 large peaches

- 1 tablespoon fresh or dried mint leaves (or 1 peppermint tea bag)

- 4 cups filtered water

- Juice of ½ lemon

Method

1. Firstly, location mint leaves or mint tea bag right into a bowl, cowl with boiling water and go away for 5-10 mins for the taste to infuse.

2. Leave till absolutely cooled.

3. De-stone and peel the peaches and mix with a small quantity of water till smooth.

4. Combine the cooled tea with the peach puree and upload lemon juice, pour right into a mason jar after which location withinside the refrigerator.

5. Drink and revel in!

Orange & Ginger Iced Tea

If warming, aromatic and citrusy liquids are your thing, then you're going to adore this iced tea. As you would possibly already know, oranges are fairly alkaline and include many residences to assist your frame detox, re-energize and stability. Ginger is great on the subject of recuperation too - it successfully treats digestive upsets and sickness, is an powerful anti-inflammatory, boosts your immune device and is likewise a first-rate alkalizer. This recipe is one of the most effective and maximum scrumptious teas on this book.

Ingredients

- 2 inches fresh ginger, cut into slices

- 1 medium orange

- 4 cups filtered water

- 1 cup iced filtered water

Method

1. Place the ginger slices right into a saucepan with the four cups of filtered water. Bring to the boil, then simmer for 10 mins.

2. Next grate the zest from the orange and squeeze the juice (in that order) and upload to the ginger and water aggregate.

3. Strain the aggregate and go away till absolutely cool.

4. Add the iced water and location withinside the refrigerator till you're equipped to revel in it.

Grapefruit & Cinnamon Iced Tea

Grapefruit is any other citrus fruit that boasts many great blessings, however because of its tart taste, lots of us don't consume a lot of the entire fruit itself. This tangy aggregate will praise the grapefruit, wake up your flavor buds, stability your pH degrees and heal your frame all on the equal time. Grapefruit is famend for its alkalizing residences, cinnamon can assist decrease your blood- sugar, lessen cravings, raise your immune device and stability your hormones, and the allspice berries upload a mild kick to the tea in addition to essential minerals and antioxidants.

Ingredients

- 2 large pink/red grapefruit

- 1 stick dried cinnamon

- ½ teaspoon whole allspice berries (optional)

- ½ cup filtered water

- Juice of ½ lemon

Method

1. Firstly, juice the grapefruit and pour right into a saucepan.

2. Add the water, cinnamon, allspice berries and lemon juice and produce to a boil.

3. Strain the aggregate and permit to cool.

4. Drink served over ice and revel in!

You also can serve this tea warm, in case you wish.

Alkalizing Bedtime Tea

For the ones instances while you need to calm down withinside the evening, soothe your worn-out frame and calm your mind, chamomile tea is perfect. But this heat tea is barely different - with the addition of alkalizing limes and sparkling detoxification apples, you'll have a barely candy but efficiently alkalizing tea to revel in. But you don't need to wait till bedtime to revel in it both. Make up a flask and take it with you to paintings for all-day calming and pH balancing benefits!

Ingredients

- 2 bags chamomile tea

- 3 fresh limes

- 1 small green apple

- 2 cups filtered water, boiling.

Method

1. Place tea baggage right into a pot and pour over the boiling water.

Leave for five mins to steep after which get rid of the baggage.

2. Meanwhile, byskip the apple thru your juicer and preserve the juice.

3. Squeeze the juice from the limes into the apple juice, and integrate with the tea.

4. Serve both heat, or cool relying at the season and your preference.

Lemon & Cayenne Alkalizing Tonic

For the ones instances you simply don't sense like ingesting down a massive glass of juice or smoothie however nevertheless need all the benefits, this small alkalizing tonic will do the trick. It's a extremely good metabolism booster this is packed complete of antioxidants, mind-healthful compounds and alkalizing enzymes. The apple cider vinegar is one of the satisfactory pH balancers out there, and cayenne will combat free-radicals, raise your mind characteristic and assist you shed any undesirable fats withinside the process.

Ingredients

- 1 lemon

- 1 teaspoon Apple Cider Vinegar

- 1/8 teaspoon cayenne

- 2 fluid ounces filtered water

- Crushed ice

Method

1. Juice the lemon and upload to a small glass, together with the relaxation of the components.

2. Top up with beaten ice (optional) and revel in!

Spicy Turmeric Alkalizing Tonic

Feeling brave? This alkalizing tonic isn't for the faint-of-heart, however this effective and effective concoction will efficiently lessen infection and go back you to pH balanced perfection in a brief and smooth way. The coconut water base includes critical electrolytes to help you to keep hydration and alkalize your frame, and the spices ginger, cayenne and turmeric will assist you shed pounds, increase a more potent immune machine, raise your cognition and preserve you feeling vibrant and energized!

Ingredients

- 3 lemons, peeled

- 2 teaspoons powdered turmeric (you can also juice fresh turmeric)

- 3 inch piece fresh ginger

- Pinch cayenne pepper

- 4 cups coconut water (or filtered water)

Method

1. Peel the lemons and upload on your juicer together with the sparkling ginger.

2. Add the lemon and ginger juice to the coconut water.

3. Next stir withinside the turmeric and cayenne pepper.

4. Pop into the refrigerator to relax after which revel in!

The Easiest Homemade Alkalizing Tonic EVER

This must be the very best selfmade alkalizing tonic ever, containing simply baking soda and filtered water. It's extraordinary for balancing your pH levels, soothing indigestion and different digestive issues, treating acne, combating cancers, or even whitening your teeth. Give this brief tonic a pass and spot what you think. A phrase of warning - these things is pretty effective so please don't devour multiple teaspoon in line with day. You might also additionally cut up measurements in 1/2 of to devour two times an afternoon in case you wish.

Ingredients

- 1 teaspoon baking soda (sodium bicarbonate)

- 8 ounces filtered water

Method

1. This one is so smooth, it's only a case of integrate and drink.

Do now no longer devour this combination with meals as it is able to intervene with digestion and belly acids.

CHAPTER 4

Quenching Vitamin Water

Have you observed nutrition water but? If now no longer, you're lamentably lacking out! They're the suitable healthy and thirst-quenching deal with for while you sense like some thing light, fruity and nutritious. Forget the ones processed-sugar cordials or chemical sweetened flavored waters - those recipes flavor notable and nourish you from the inner out.

Of course, they assist preserve you hydrated and rebalance your pH levels, and throw in an entire load greater benefits; which includes soothing your digestive machine, boosting your immune machine, recuperation your skin, assisting you to shed pounds and additionally assisting to preserve cancer, Alzheimer's sickness and diabetes at bay.

Enjoy them at any time of the day, any day of the week and irrespective of wherein you are. Simply blend up a massive jug of your favourite infusion and take it together with you anyplace you pass, sipping, recuperation and feeding each mobileular on your frame. Here are my pinnacle 3 blends of all time.

Mint & Lemongrass Vitamin Water

Could your digestive machine do with a assisting hand? This nutrition water may want to nicely be your answer. The pineapple will useful resource in pH stability and soothe your digestive tract, the lemongrass is notable for detoxing and treating tummy aches, and the sparkling ginger will assist save you illness, raise your immune machine and heat you from head to toe.

Ingredients

- 1 cup pineapple
- Small handful fresh mint (to taste)
- 3 inches fresh ginger
- 1 inch fresh lemongrass
- 1 liter filtered water
- Juice of ½ lemon

Method

1. Place ginger and mint in a small bowl and muddle (overwhelm gently) with the lower back of a spoon or with a muddler.

2. Next upload the pineapple chunks and repeat the process.

3. Then throw all the components right into a massive glass jar or chrome steel bottle and pinnacle up with the water.

4. Place into your refrigerator for 4-eight hours to infuse, then revel in!

Ultimate Citrus Vitamin Water

If you've examine the relaxation of this book, you'll recognize why I'm so enthusiastic about citrus end result. They are, definitely one of the first-class methods to stability your physical pH levels, as they may be effective, less expensive and scrumptious too.

This citrus nutrition water is 'ultimate' for a superb reason - it incorporates lots of citrus end result to provide a drink packed complete of nutrients, antioxidants and different recovery characteristics too. Feel loose to feature your very own citrus additions to customize this scrumptious nutrition infusion.

Ingredients

- 1 medium grapefruit
- 1 orange, thinly sliced
- ½ lemon, thinly sliced
- ½ lime, thinly sliced
- Juice of ½ lemon
- 1 liter filtered water

Method

1. Juice the grapefruit and lemon, and upload to a huge glass jar or chrome steel bottle.

2. Add the slices of citrus fruit and pinnacle up with the filtered water.

3. Replace the lid and depart to take a seat down and infuse withinside the refrigerator for 4-eight hours.

4. Drink and enjoy!

Very Berry Vitamin Water

This nutrition water captures the alkalizing and nourishing residences of berries, provides a great dose of electrolyte-wealthy coconut water, packs in nutrient- wealthy spirulina strength and provides a sprint of lemon juice to create the first-class alkalizing berry beverage! Perfect for rebalancing your pH levels, boosting your immune system, regaining your electricity and recuperating from illness.

Ingredients

- 1 cup fresh coconut water
-

- ○ 1/2 cup raspberries
- • 1/2 cup blackberries
- • 1 teaspoon spirulina powder
- • 1 liter filtered water
- • Juice of ½ lemon

Method

1. Place the berries right into a small bowl and pour over a number of the coconut water. Muddle (lightly crush).

2. Add the relaxation of the ingredients, taking care to stir the spirulina powder into the water well.

3. Top up with filtered water, pour into a pitcher jar or bottle, and depart to take a seat down withinside the refrigerator for 4-eight hours.

4. Drink and enjoy!

Printed in Great Britain
by Amazon

34511657R00094